Claiming Your Inner Gifts

To Robyn —

Happy Birthday, Friend!

i Hope this is an Amazing
Year For you!

All love,
Jen

Claiming Your Inner Gifts

The Comprehensive Study of Master Reiki

Mastering Your Life and Reiki

Marnie Vincolisi

This book is not intended as a substitute for the medical recommendations of physicians or other health-care providers. Rather, it is intended to offer alternative information to help the reader cooperate with physicians and health professionals in a mutual quest for optimal well-being and a better understanding of self.

Published by Light Internal
Littleton, Colorado
www.lightinternal.com

Book covers design by Rich Allen

ISBN 978-0-9823732-2-4

Dedication

This book is dedicated to the master who lies dormant within all of us.
May this book inspire you to step into your power and claim your greatness.

May I remind you that everything you read between the pages of this book is to satisfy your analytical mind. Once that is accomplished, let go of the information and know that you already embody the manifestation of all your hopes, dreams and desires. You have the ability to master whatever you put your mind to and you have the assistance of a myriad of light beings who are listening and ready to respond to your request. I am here to make you aware that you already walk with these beings in the higher dimensions every day and you can easily awaken this knowledge. I support you in your travels through the realms of light.

Marnie Vincolisi

Table of Contents

Introduction

When you make the commitment to become a Reiki master you are telling the Universe you are ready for major changes to occur in every aspect of your life. This is not a vow to take lightly because at this level the attunement given will be a clearing at the soul level. This will allow you to work directly with the soul of your client. And as in all levels of Reiki when we give Reiki we get Reiki. With that in mind, when you are helping your client heal at the soul level you will receive a deep soul healing as well, every time you practice Reiki. This is what will really allow your spirit to soar.

In first degree Reiki it is suggested to ask permission to give Reiki to another. This honors the free will of the client as they always have permission to refuse the service. Once a practitioner becomes a master of Reiki they no longer need to follow this rule completely. Respect is always given to the client and the choices they make but at this level of Reiki because you are working with the soul of the client, permission is almost always granted by their soul.

Reiki is a non-invasive practice; the energy is directed to the part of the body which is in the most need. This course is guided by the higher self of the client but when a master stands by their side supporting them it allows the process to touch deeper core issues. For this reason it is important for the master to continue their exercise of administering self Reiki. The phrase "Physician heal thy self" certainly applies. Reiki is pure divine love; it can soften the hardest soul and enlighten the greatest skeptic. If the master's heart is not full to overflowing with love, they could take on the doubt and fear of others thus lessening the work performed. When the master takes time to open to the love around them by applying self Reiki, their stance in this practice becomes unwavering.

The Light Internal system of Reiki includes the practice of both traditional and nontraditional Reiki. This allows the student an extensive education so that they can find and then embody their true healing abilities. The student may step into their true calling, unencumbered by individual opinions outside of their own. The following teachings are guidelines to be followed and then released, revealing how Reiki works for each particular healer, opening them to the gifts they hold within themselves.

Once you receive your attunement know that whether you feel the energy or not, it is there working for you. There will be times when the force is quite unmistakable and yet other times when there is no sensation. When I was first attuned to Reiki master level, I cannot say I felt the energy of the symbols immediately. It took me some time to sense what was happening in my energy field but I did notice major changes in my life. This was my signal I was transforming, yet I did not always sense it in my hands when I applied Reiki.

The first major change I noticed was that I had the strength to leave a religious group which was negating my power. I was able to open my heart and I began a spiritual relationship with my own divine self, unencumbered by religious dogma. I created an entirely new business which was supportive of my creative nature and it placed me on a new enlightened path. So during your training don't think just because you do not "feel" what you think you "should feel" that your Reiki attunement is not working. Reiki always works.

Reiki is a full time job, or rather; a gift that is shared all the time. A job is often something you have to do and channeling Reiki is something you want to do because it is such a natural way of being. Once you are touched by Reiki the desire to give it to others often becomes very prevalent. Reiki is always flowing through the eyes of the master, out through their aura, filling a room, and flowing to all who are near. The Universal life force of Reiki is pure love and through that love, others feel calm. When a master walks into a room, the vibration of the room rises because of the high frequency of the master. The master is always radiating Reiki, which is pure love; it can't be avoided. The more attention put towards Reiki, the higher the vibration becomes in and around the master and it starts making a difference in every facet of their life and those in their life. It is by conscious awareness that these changes are ever increasing.

After your master attunement, observe how your life is changing. What is empowering you, how are you reacting to others and how are you claiming your gifts? This will be your message that you are now in the realm of master. Don't look back for change a week or a month ago; look back six months ago or even a year ago. Is life smoother, gentler, easier? Are people responding differently to you? Do you find yourself less aggravated and upset? Have you seen old situations in a new light? Can you flow with life as difficulties are handed to you? Have relationships dispersed which had turmoil? Did they dissolve without struggle?

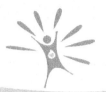

The beauty of Reiki comes from its simplicity. Aside from the practice of applying Reiki to one self a few times a week, there is really nothing that needs to be done other than use it. Give it to those in your life, direct it to strangers you pass on the street, to the cars as they pass on the highway, an ambulance, hearse or political figure. You may have already found yourself doing this as the Reiki attunements open you to becoming aware of the world around you and the love of Reiki makes you want to help others. There is no place for others to hide for now you can see behind the veil they have drawn about themselves and you can quickly see who is in need of love. And that would be everyone.

Reiki channels the purest form of love. It holds no judgment and once it is given to another the master is released from the responsibility of how the Reiki will proceed. It will be guided by the higher self of the recipient and enter their heart and soul. The Reiki master's job is to draw to themselves the ones who will be open to receiving this divine light. The synchronicities which begin to occur are phenomenal. A day begins and you think it will be just like any other day and soon the tide turns and you become the observer of how Reiki is moving you towards your true path in life.

There are many ways to develop intuitive skills, and having a variety of methods to approach these abilities will be beneficial to the practitioner as well as the client. Over time you will be presented with many opportunities to fine tune the way you assist the people who will step into your life. Not all will be clients, some will be business associates, friends or just ones who pass by and you will apply a quick method you have learned to help them. Your energy as a master will radiate out from your physical presence and be apparent to some on a conscious level and some will respond on a subconscious level. But nonetheless, many will respond to your higher vibration. Mankind is in need of the light which you now carry. Be aware, when you acknowledge you hold a light within you that that is all that is required. You will not need to make any special adjustments to send it out to others. It happens automatically.

There are many techniques tucked away in the pages of this book but they are not really necessary to transform yourself or others. Each process is designed to appease the conscious mind, that part of your psychic which wants to be fed intellectual information. This is your left brain trying to figure out why hands on healing makes one feel better. It wants to know how the intuitive process works and why it does not perform the same all the time.

For this aspect of your brain I give you numerous Life Tools. They will give you easy step by step ways to appease the inquisitive left brain. Once that is accomplished, at the point where your brain is filled with what it thinks is necessary information, you may forget all you have learned. The way true change occurs is when one can let go of the process and accept that change has already happened. This is when the practitioner has stepped into a place of no space, no time - the quantum field of unlimited possibilities. There are very few people who have not been in this space at one time. In this place everything in life just flows without effort.

Recall a time when this happened for you. It could be when you first fell in love, sometime in high school when you were participating in a school event such as sports or a play or an experience you have had in the business arena. At that time it took no effort to accomplish your goals. That is the time I am referencing. By applying the processes in this book you will feed your left brain so you may then stop the analytical chatter and slip into this indescribable place where all things are possible. I invite you to sit back and fill your left brain with understandable concepts and then let it all dissolve as you accept yourself as master of your life and step into the field which cannot be described, only felt.

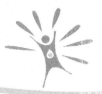

Chapter 1

Symbols

The Reiki symbols are given as a tool to assist not only in the process of applying Reiki during treatments but in everyday situations as well. There are a myriad of choices we can make in any given moment; some will advance us on a perceived path while others will throw us off balance for a time. The Reiki symbols can help to energize our decisions while making the right path more apparent.

The symbols were never meant to be an absolute. When they are first presented to a student they are to be practiced so the practitioner will discover how the symbols work with their clients and in various situations. At times the symbols will be drawn in the air and other times they may only require the intent to call in their power. The process will be different for each individual who applies them. Once these discoveries are made the symbols will be used with the frequency decided by the wisdom of the practitioner.

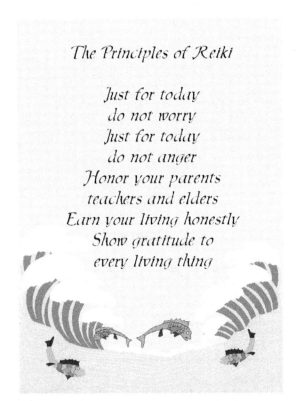

The Principles of Reiki

Just for today
do not worry
Just for today
do not anger
Honor your parents
teachers and elders
Earn your living honestly
Show gratitude to
every living thing

There are a few translations of the Principles of Reiki and this one has a focus upon honoring teachers. The statement, "honor your parents, teachers and elders" is from traditional Reiki training. The master teacher was always put in the highest regard, sometimes to the invalidation of the students themselves. The Light Internal system teaches the initiates to honor themselves as well as their instructors. Society has shown us to honor everyone else but ourselves, and yet if we do not fully love and respect ourselves, it becomes difficult to honor others. There can be resentment in honoring another when you do not honor yourself first. The accolades in others are revealed when you claim them within yourself. The beauty of honoring other masters is that you will then have claimed their qualities within yourself, thus empowering you with the statement. Honor your parents, teachers and elders," rather than giving your power away to another.

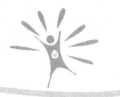

As the student practices using Reiki along with the support of the symbols they will find many uses not found printed in books. It is helpful to keep a group of Reiki practitioners close at hand so they can share experiences and thus have an opportunity to learn from each other. This practice will keep the experience of Reiki growing and validated. There is no limit to what can be obtained by applying the love of Reiki every day to everyone.

There are 4 traditional symbols which are the original Reiki symbols used by the original grand masters of Reiki: Dr. Mikao Usui, Dr. Chujiro Hayashi and Hawayo Takata. These traditional symbols are Cho-Ku-Rei, Sei-He-Ki, Hon-Sha-Ze-Sho-Nen and Dai-Ko-Myo. The other symbols, Cho-Ku-Ret, Ran-Sei Fire Serpent and Modern Dai-Ko-Mio are nontraditional symbols and were never used by the masters who lived in the early 1900s. This does not diminish their power and ability to assist in the application of Reiki and in life situations.

Cho-Ku-Rei in its simplicity can advance the student because there are so many times just calling in the power and love of Reiki can change the course of a situation that appears to have gone wrong. There is a quality in it which creates a very strong grounding effect. Anchoring the energy to the earth will assist the practitioner to channel not only healing love from the cosmos but nurturing love from the earth as well. Seeing we are earth bound beings, this grounding effect will make healing attributes stronger than before. Grounding is a natural part of our anatomy, for every element which is found in the earth can also be found in our body as well. So connecting to the earth is like going home. It can create a beautiful bubble of love that when used can radiate such peace and confidence that things automatically go the right way. It becomes quite fun to apply this energy throughout the day.

Sei-He-Ki when blended with the energy of an attuned Reiki Master will gently bring to the fore front the emotional issues which have held the client back in the past. Because the master has the gift to work with the soul of the client, the deepest healing can occur. All fear and concerns should be dispersed when the question arises in your mind, "Am I going to bring in more emotions than the client can handle?"

Remember: the client will not open to a recollection they cannot manage; their higher self is always guiding the process. If an issue arises the client is ready to face it and is supported in the process.

Hon-Sha-Ze-Sho-Nen is the symbol of movement. It holds no healing qualities of its own yet its power is unsurpassed. Doors will open when the master can conceptualize, that this symbol can do more than move healing energy across the miles. By having the intent to direct the healing into the dimensions of time and space, the master can resolve core issues. These elements of time can be in the past, present, future or parallel realities.

The only way Hon-Sha-Ze-Sho-Nen can be used is with the mind. The thought of how and where it travels is a mindful act. Hence this symbol is directly connected to the mental body. To move the healing light to heal old situations it will be asked to travel into the past. It can gain entrance to the Akashic records which are an etheric database of everything which has occurred in a soul's existence whether they were in a body or in the spirit realm. There are times when accessing this knowledge can shed a light on present day issues. When there is a desire to create support for future events this symbol will carry the intent of Reiki love into the future. In present time it will move the energy across the room, miles or into the spiritual, mental or emotional bodies of the client.

In parallel time frames incidents are happening at the same time as present-day situations but in different dimensions. Science has described this phenomenon as the string theory. In the past scientists claimed no two objects could occupy the same space at the same time. They have now proven that indeed two objects can occupy the same space at the same time only if they are in alternate dimensions. This paradox can also happen within the mental and emotional body. By directing Reiki into all timeframes, the love of Reiki will access the parallel aspects of the client's psyche as well, which will clear issues deep within the core of the client's entire being. The master attunement will open the intuition of the initiate so these concepts are seen, felt and understood, thus allowing them to greatly assist their clients in understanding how they are clearing issues.

Dai-Ko-Myo connects to the highest level of Reiki and houses the qualities of all of the traditional symbols. If the master desires, this could be the only symbol they ever will use again. When the student is attuned to Dai-Ko-Myo they may more quickly gain access to the soul of the client to assist them at the deepest core level.

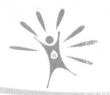

Symbols and Our Energy Bodies

Each of the four traditional symbols resonates with the four physical and etheric bodies. When you recall the cleanse you experienced with each Reiki attunement it becomes easy to remember the line-up of the symbols to the body. First degree Reiki holds a physical opening to the Reiki energy and it is often felt in the body during the cleansing process. The initiate could feel tired, energized, queasy or headachy. Because Cho-Ku-Rei is so grounding it makes sense that it will be connected to the physical body. The second degree of Reiki introduces the student to the mental and emotional symbol and will often bring emotions to the surface during the cleansing period. Therefore Sei-He-Kei is the symbol associated with the emotional body. Hon-Sha-Ze-Sho-Nen can only be sent by through the thought process so it will be associated with the mind. The attunement cleanse often also awakens the soul of the initiate and so Dai-Ko-Myo will be the symbol which connects to the soul.

1. The physical body attunes to Cho-Ku-Rei.

    1st degree attunement cleanse usually affects the physical form.
2. The emotional body will be associated with Sei-He-Ki.

    2nd degree attunement cleanse often affects the emotional body.
3. The mental body touches Hon-Sha-Ze-Sho-Nen.

    The movement of Reiki with this symbol is directed by the thoughts in the mind; therefore this symbol is connected to the mental body.
4. The spiritual body will correlate with Dai-Ko-Myo.

    3rd degree attunement cleanse clears the spiritual body for a soul-to-soul connection with the client, creating advanced healings.

The following chart is a quick reference of all the Reiki symbols. It is a review of the symbols given in first and second degree Reiki as well as the new master symbols which the master will be attuned to in third or master degree Reiki.

Cho-Ku-Rei

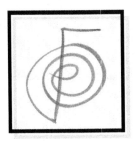

* Power symbol, strongest for physical healing and protection.
* Seals in a room and clears out negative energy.
* Anchors and grounds the practitioner and the client.

Sei-He-Ki

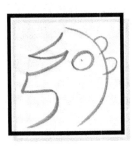

* Mental and emotional symbol.
* Clears at the core level of an issue.
* Brings mental and emotional problems to the surface.
* Opens new perspectives.
* Releases spirit attachments.

Hon-Sha-Ze-Sho-Nen

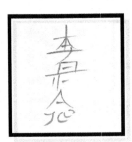

* The vehicle on which Reiki moves.
* Directs Reiki across dimensions of time and space.
* May be sent into the past or the future.
* May be used to access Akashic records.

Ran-Sei

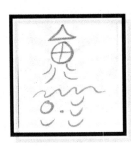

* Creates physical balance and harmony.
* Develops balance for sports, dancing, art projects.
* Supports the lymphatic system.
* Strengthens the immune system.
* Helps AIDS, HIV and cancer patients.

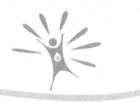

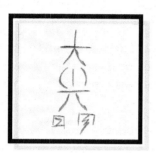
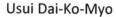

Usui Dai-Ko-Myo
* Traditional master symbol dating from the early 1900s.
* Channels the highest Reiki energy.
* Represents all traditional symbols.

Modern Dai-Ko-Mio
* Activated in the 1980s.
* Equal power to traditional symbol.
* Contains all the Reiki symbols within it.
* Reflects and honors the feminine.

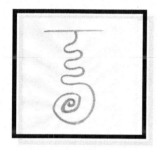

Fire Serpent
* Very strong grounding energy.
* Use at the end of a treatment to anchor healing.

Cho-Ku-Ret
* Empowers only objects.
* Use on musical instruments or sporting equipment.

Qualities of the Reiki Symbols

This review is to help you organize all the symbols taught in Reiki in one concise place. Details for each symbol are contained in the second level of Reiki or on the following pages. Use this as a quick reference to refresh your memory on each individual image.

1. Cho-Ku-Rei – traditional
    a. Activates the power of Reiki and the practitioner.
    b. Brings physical healing to a direct place.
    c. Seals any room or area in love.
    d. Clears rooms of negativity and quickly raises the vibration.
    e. Supports grounding of the practitioner, client or space.

2. Sei-He-Ki - traditional
    a. For mental and emotional balance.
    b. Floats the original cause of the disturbance to the surface.
    c. Brings spiritual meaning to emotional distress.
    d. Calls in angels and other divine assistance.
    e. Aligns the upper chakras.
    f. Releases spirit attachments.
    g. Balances and heals relationships; heals fear, depression or anger.
    h. Promotes will power to release addictions.
    i. Improves memory and helps to find lost items.
    j. Empowers affirmations.

3. Hon-Sha-Ze-Sho-Nen - traditional
    a. This symbol has no healing qualities; it is merely a vehicle to move the energy through space and time.
    b. Directs healing across over the miles as well as dimensions of time: past, present and future.
    c. Sends Reiki into future events for personal and business needs.
    d. Aids in medical procedures by sending love to all involved.
    e. Moves into the past to heal previous events or old patterns.

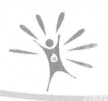

    f.   It allows Reiki to go to the original core issue in all dimensions; past present, future and, if directed so into parallel dimensions as well.

    g.   Gains entrance into Akashic records which can clear vows of poverty, religious contracts and the like. These records describe the Karmic goals, debts, contracts and life purpose of the soul.

4. Ran-Sei – nontraditional

    a.   Creates physical balance and harmony on the physical level.

    b.   Helps to clean toxins out of the lymphatic system.

    c.   Assists AIDS, HIV and cancer patients.

    d.   Strengthens the immune system.

    e.   Brings balance to objects with their alignment to the body as in sports equipment (skis, golf clubs, skates.)

5. Fire Serpent - Tibetan, nontraditional

    a.   Power booster like Cho-Ku-Rei, but much stronger.

    b.   Use at the end of a treatment to anchor the client's energy to the earth.

6. Cho-Ku-Ret - nontraditional

    a.   Use on inanimate objects.

    b.   Use on musical instruments, art brushes, sports equipment, anything which requires balance to use.

Ran Sei

Nontraditional Symbol

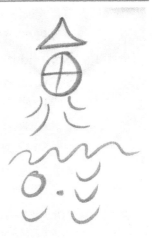

Ran-Sei is not one of the original symbols taught by Usui or Takata therefore it is a nontraditional symbol. It still holds an ability to balance energies when used while channeling Ran-Sei but is not a symbol which will always be used at the beginning of a treatment. Use it at your discretion when you need to support the lymphatic system or strengthen the immune system. It can balance the entire physical body, as well as the etheric bodies: spiritual, mental and emotional. It can align the yin and yang energies of the body which are the masculine and the feminine polarities. Once applied it opens the individual to create a marriage of the divine aspects of these forces. Because it holds the quality of balance it can be used on objects and how they align with the body in sports, art or play.

There is a geometric flow to this symbol as it balances from left to right and from male to female. The direction of the lines are not congruent, they switch back and forth from right to left and up and down which reflects balance. Observe that the top of the image is made of straight lines which are representative of male energy while the feminine curves are seen in the lower part of the image. When the drawing is fully complete one can see the balance it creates as it honors the differences of the male and female while simultaneously joining them. The center wave line reflects water, which holds the emotions. The differences become apparent from the beginning to the end of the symbol. In the activation of this balance is how the body regains its health.

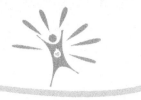

Drawing Ran-Sei

The effects from activating the energy of Ran-Sei:

- Creates balance and harmony on the physical level.
- Cleanses the lymphatic system.
- Strengthens the immune system.
- Assists AIDS, HIV and cancer patients.
- Balances inanimate objects.

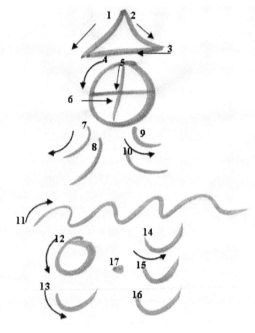

   Follow the arrows and notice how the direction of the first two lines appears as energy flowing from the divine down from the peak of the triangle over the entire symbol. The circle can be seen as a representation of the earth because movement #4, is drawn counterclockwise and the center cross, #5 and #6, honors the four directions; north, south, east and west. The practice of walking counterclockwise during ceremonies and showing respect to the four directions has been used by indigenous people for eons of time, thus acknowledging their love and respect for earth. #7 to #10 is the flow from the divine masculine down to the curvy existence of feminine reflected at the bottom of this symbol.

   #11 flows like water which is often signifies emotion which is a female trait and #12 drawn counterclockwise as the circle before. #17 is the final touch, the period at the end of a sentence and the energy which pushes the intent of this symbol out into the Universe where it will be received and used for the highest purpose for all concerned.

   Even within the drawing of this symbol one can detect balance in its movement. Unlike Hon Sha Ze Sho Nen where all lines are drawn from top to bottom and from left to right, Ran-Sei switches back and forth in every direction It begins by moving down at #1 and #2 and then #3 is from right to left, yet #6 changes and moves from left to right. #7 to #10 move down while #13 to #16 move up. The change in directions is what gives this symbol its balance visually and supports the intent of balance.

 Remember: Nothing is stronger than your intent. Honor each symbol and draw it to the best of your ability but be assured, it is your intent which makes it work, not your accuracy of its design.

Balancing the Masculine and Feminine

When in a good mental state we are a balance between both our masculine and feminine elements, no matter what gender we have embodied. These opposite parts of us can hold their individuality as they support and share their differences in our bodies. Ran-Sei can help in stabilizing these attributes. To become familiar with, balance and obtain information from your opposite gender, you may draw Ran-Sei as you enter into a meditation with the intent to greet the divine aspect of your masculine and feminine self.

Example: I set aside a time to explore how my male and female aspects might present themselves to me. I was not in a relationship at the time and I was curious to see what these divine aspects were about. I wanted to notice if a visit with them might give me an insight into my relationship with men.

Within the stillness of my mind I found, much to my surprise my male and female not paying much attention to each other. They were not talking or even looking at each other. They were standing back to back, apparently content to look out over the cosmos without any interaction with each other. I did not feel this was out of balance but because I desired a relationship with a man I invited them to turn and face each other. They completed my request and as I watched them I could see that was enough movement for the time and my meditation ended.

The next week I once again looked upon them and this time I spent more time during my contemplation observing and instructing them to take the next step. I had them embrace each other and in that moment I felt a beautiful energy rain down upon my

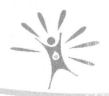

physical body. I watched them and it did not take long for them to begin dancing in the sky. After this meditation I felt more at peace about my current situation. I do not recall how long it was till I met a man on the physical plane to dance with, but the peace that came from this encounter allowed the element of time not to matter. The serenity came in knowing I could interact with these aspects of myself and appease my active mind which always wants to do something to push change. In this way I did not feel I had to do anything physically, for my divine was balanced.

 Remember: We are human beings, not human doings - *Neale Donald Walsch*

This reminder instructs us to stop trying to make things happen, instead go with the flow. Then trust that the Universe will provide for our necessities.

 Life Tool: Meeting your Divine Male and Female

1.	Set the intent that you will become familiar with the divine male and female aspects of yourself.
2.	Take three long deep breaths and with each breath allow your mind to become silent. Then each and every muscle in your body will relax.
3.	Drop into your center and notice if this core space is in your heart or a chakra. It could also be a still feeling which has no location and you cannot describe it.
4.	Relax in this quiet place for a few minutes and when you are ready, imagine moving above your head.
5.	Direct your attention to the area where your divine masculine and feminine reside. Do not impose a particular place to your mind, let it happen naturally.
6.	Once you reach the place where you can see this dual aspect of yourself observe how high you are above your body. As you look around can you see the earth, the sky or the cosmos?

7.	Look upon the duality of your divine self and ask any questions you might have and allow their knowledge to enlighten you.
8.	You are the creator of this part of yourself, so you may redirect, change or manage how they interplay with each other. Make this fun rather than control.
9.	When you feel your visit is complete float back into your body and know you can observe, redirect and converse with them at any future time of your choosing.

Harmony Supporting the Immune System

When the body is reflecting ill health often the lymphatic system is in overload as it tries to cleanse the body of the inhibitors, yet it is unable to keep up with the pace. This can be true with cancer, AIDS, HIV and even colds and flu. Ran-Sei in its balancing qualities will assist in opening and clearing the lymphatic system so it can work at the capacity required for optimum health. In this way the immune system is strengthened.

When a patient is informed they have contacted a life-threatening disease the mind can begin to create a scenario which can spin more destructive energy into the body and add to the imbalance created by the disease. In order to combat this mental spiral a new image can be conjured up to heal the body so the dis-ease has less hold on the mind and body of the individual.

Once this picture is created, one can readjust the imbalances within their conscious and subconscious mind. This can be accomplished by imagining the body as a symphony and when it is in harmony, it is healthy and all the organs and cells will vibrate to the music held within. When the body displays ill health the music can be off key and/or the instruments out of tune. During a Reiki treatment you may direct the client to hold the image of harmony in each cell of their body. Reiki will place the individual into their subconscious mind where a new story can be constructed and these changes can become permanent.

The body is an incredible machine which can be seen as a symphony. It is synchronized at every level, becoming clear about this process will allow the cells begin to

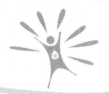

change into healthier cells. It has been said that we need to live in harmony, but did you ever think of that harmony being within every cell of your body? In music harmony is not being the same as another note but the blending of different tones into a pleasing arrangement. Each note sounds different yet the distance they hold from each other creates the simplicity of its beautiful sound. I learned the true meaning of harmony one summer day in the Rocky Mountains.

Example: I was on a tour with my healing buddies in search of spiritual places in and around Colorado. We ventured to a church in New Mexico which was known for healing the lame. Santuario Chimayo was just outside of Taos. I soon would find this church had more in store for me than I had imagined.

It was all very synchronistic because when we arrived at this church it was just as high mass began. We sat in the pews with the local people and when it came time for communion I was acquainted with the element of harmony. A procession began as the parishioners sang as they walked up to the altar. One woman walked by me and was singing beautifully and her voice stood out. I realized she was not singing the same notes as the others, she was singing in harmony. At that point I realized what harmony really reflected. It is being different than anyone else, even standing out, but still within the balance of others while complementing who and what they are.

So many times we try to fit in with a group, thinking we need to be like them. Fortunately as we mature we begin to understand that we do not have to conform to be accepted; in fact our differences will create the harmony needed for peace and love within the family, business or personal unit. If we were all the same notes there would be no song.

In that respect let us look at cancer in this way: energetically the cancer cells have formed a hard shell around themselves for protection. The protection is required to shield the individual from stress, emotional pain or lack of love. Because of this layer, they do not hear the music of their body's symphony therefore they are not in resonance with the other cells. They grow rapidly because of this disconnection and are out of sync with the entire body system. Rather than eliminate these cells, ask the client to send love to them and awaken them so they may once again be aligned to the music held within the healthy cells.

Concentrate on one cell and then ask it to replicate throughout the body. This will save time and the process can be interesting and empowering to observe. When the client can see the change they have made within their body the entire process takes on the semblance of reality. This will give them power to know they can make changes within their body and their life. Once they establish love in the cells of the body their physical world will begin to, reflect the same.

Ran-Sei, if directed, will open the tough shell around the cancer cell so it will be connected with the normal cells. The unhealthy cells can then hear the harmonious music in the body and mimic the healthy tones and cease to grow out of control. This brings balance back to the physical form, while giving the patient a loving way to approach this fearful dis-ease.

Balancing Objects with Ran-Sei

Ran-Sei can also be used on inanimate objects to assist in their balance and accuracy. Use it for sports and while playing musical instruments. Apply Ran-Sei and discover its unlimited uses. Use it on golf clubs, roller blades, skis, dancing, pottery throwing, yoga and music in all forms. This list can be expanded according to the interest of yourself and your clients.

Example: One of my students was a piano teacher most of her life and was now in her 70s. She learned Reiki and began to apply this symbol on the piano and music before the children arrived for their lessons. She was pleased to announce their nervousness diminished and the activity of merely hitting the keys changed into the flow of playing music.

Another Reiki practitioner used Ran-Sei not only on her golf clubs but on the ball as well. This helped her as the athlete and the ball stay on course.

Anyone who has attempted pottery as a hobby soon discovers if you are not centered and balanced, the potter's wheel will reflect this lack of symmetry. When sitting at the wheel before turning it on, still your thoughts, imagine Ran-Sei in your mind's eye, ground your energy to the earth and then begin working the mud.

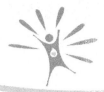

As you can see, nontraditional symbols can be quite helpful in your everyday life, thus supporting the idea that Reiki is not just for healing. It is designed to use daily for harmony, balance and love, during work and play.

Fire Serpent

Nontraditional Tibetan Symbol

The Fire Serpent is another nontraditional symbol but this one can be substituted for the power symbol at the end of the treatment and used at other times during the day. It looks like Cho-Ku-Rei and has a similar energy. The difference is that it has an amazing grounding effect especially when it is drawn over the body. One can feel how it pulls the entire body to the earth as it anchors it.

 Remember: Your healing attributes will be stronger if you simultaneously connect to the earth as well as drawing from the cosmos.

To recall how to draw this image think of Cho-Ku-Rei and extend the swirl from the downward line to the bottom and take that downward line and make it squiggle back and forth. Compare the two symbols to the side.

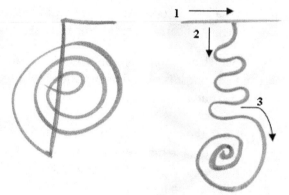

Cho-Ku-Rei   Fire Serpent

There is an explanation for what the lines represent on many of the symbols. The curved lines at the bottom the Cho-Ku-Rei and Fire Serpent show the grounding connection to the earth. These swirls have been seen drawn in caves and used in art work by indigenous people for eons of time. This reflects the relationship of tribes of old and the earth. This spiral of energy is also part of nature for this twirl can be seen in flowers, rams horns, sea shells and even out to the cosmos in the spin of the galaxy. This is what gives these grounding symbols their amazing power for they connect to the earth and sky simultaneously which is also what happens when one channels Reiki.

When using Fire Serpent over a client's body, place the swirl at the bottom of their feet, to ground the healing energy of the treatment into the earth. This will anchor the effects of the healing into their everyday affairs with a subtle grounding effect. Mention to the client that Reiki will continue to assist them for three days after their session so they will watch for the changes. This will assist them to become a conscious part of their own healing. Their observations will deepen the effect of the session as they can see the inevitable changes in their mind and body.

Using Fire Serpent at the end of a treatment will secure the healing work in all four bodies: physical, mental, emotional and spiritual. With the connections of these bodies to the earth there is a greater opportunity to fully integrate their healing process. This promotes the healing of core issues, so that old patterns are not repeated.

To find out which grounding symbol you prefer, draw them on your body. Start with Cho-Ku-Rei and imagine it is placed over both of your feet and observe the grounding effect.

- Imagine the top line moving across the toes.
- The center line moves down the foot and stops at the instep or center of the foot; this is the location of the foot chakra.
- At that point see the swirl not only moving around the chakra but also dropping into the earth to anchor the energies.
- Observe how this feels; often it feels as if you cannot move your feet from the place you are standing.

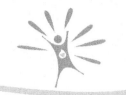

Now draw Fire Serpent according to the image presented. The straight line travels across from one hip to the other. The squiggle line moves down each leg and the swirl lands at the feet and flows into the earth as with Cho-Ku-Rei. Compare and see if you notice a difference between the two symbols. Often the awareness is that Fire Serpent grounds the entire body while Cho-Ku-Rei anchors more at the feet.

To Embody Fire Serpent

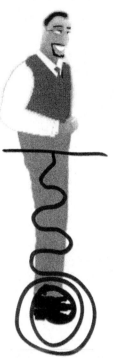

- Place the top line at the hip.
- The spiral descends down each leg for super grounding.
- The swirl is at the feet.
- This grounds Reiki to the earth.

By making your own comparisons you will fine tune your intuitive skills so that you will know what blends with your healing energy. Too often we can be swayed by the opinions of others and the media (this even includes the metaphysical media). There is always a new class, a different instructor or newly channeled information which implies that "this is the way to true spiritual healing." Do not even let the information contained in this book be an absolute. Use the knowledge as a guide line and construct your special healing talents from there.

Learn to listen to the inner feelings in your heart before you ask another their opinion about the information being presented. Remember to always first stop and check within yourself before you validate information coming from outside channels. This practice will increase your ability to discern what will be the best action for you to take for yourself or a client. Then, when opportunities arise, you will be skilled and confident to make a decision which best suits your energetic frequency. This is the mark of a true master.

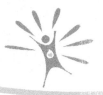

Chapter 2

Master Symbols

There are numerous master symbols which have been passed down throughout the various Reiki lineages. The initiate will find they will be guided to the master who attunes to the symbol which resonates with the student's energy. The Light Internal system of Reiki honors the unique differences in each individual; therefore not one, but *all* the master symbols are included in this practice. This allows the student to locate the symbol which resonates closest to their personal vibration which empowers them as a master.

The spelling of the master symbols varies, yet no one spelling is connected to any specific symbol. The varieties are as follows:

- Dai-Ko-Myo
- Dai-Ko-Mio
- Dai-Ku-Myo
- Dai-Koo-Myo

They may be pronounced Dai-Koo-Mio with a long "o" or Dai-Ku-Mio with a short "o". The "y" in "Myo" can be articulated with a long or short "y", being "eeee" or "iiiiii." The choice is yours. I will be using Mio in the traditional symbols and Myo for the nontraditional modern symbols. Remember that the spelling is interchangeable with all the master symbols.

As master, you have the opportunity to decide which will be your symbol of choice and this preference may change over time. I began my practice by using the Modern Dai-Ko-Myo but over the years have found the Tibetan Dai-Ko-Myo more suited to my energy. Instruction is given on how to physically embody each symbol so you may know in your cellular structure which symbol resonates with you at any given time. You will then sense when it is time to move to another symbol or stay with the original one you picked.

Over time, the preferred symbol may change as the student transforms. All master symbols have equal power; one is not stronger than another. All the master symbols are included in this Reiki master system so that the student, soon to be master, can make their own decision as to which symbol is right for them, without the influence of their master teacher. The desire to use a particular master symbol may become different as the needs of a client change and the energy of the master is raised and altered. The ability to be more aware of everything in our surroundings is one of the gifts of Reiki; this allows the initiate to be open to their ever changing world and how they resonate within it. The various choices of the master symbols given, permit the student to become more responsive to the current situation of their client and thus to use the appropriate symbol.

In sacred geometry, straight lines are representative of the male, while curved lines hold the gender of the feminine. When looking at the physical female form, one notices that it curves while the male is very linear in body and often in mind. Male energy can be more left brain, exact, precise and orderly, while the female energy is more right brain, intuitive and flowing. These, of course, are generalizations and not made to be absolute. It is the blending of these energies in a partnership which makes it balanced and also challenging. This allows us to keep in mind that even during turmoil, all is in divine order.

The master symbols which were activated in the early 1900s have male energy, which are revealed in their straight lines. During that time most spiritual practices were guided by gurus and wise beings with power, who were almost always male. Since that time, the vibration of the earth and those who inhabit her has risen. The ones who are now walking

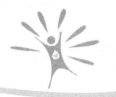

and seeking a spiritual path, who have embodied from the late 1940s on, are gurus in their own right. They are self-empowered and do not need the constant attention of a master as they journey upward in life. I would say that you, who read this book, are of that higher vibration which gives you the power to find your own path, transcend the limitations of this earthly plane, and if you desire, assist others to do so as well.

The new master symbols which have come in since the 1980s are female in their origin, as seen by the curved lines. They guide us to embody the pure love of Reiki and other high vibrational frequencies. Work with the various master symbols and see if you notice any difference in their effects either in the energy you channel or in the response of your client.

Example: The early Dai-Ko-Mio can be used when assessing information for an elderly client who has lived in the early 1900s. This symbol could also apply to a teenage client who has lived a past life in the 1900s and has now returned to clear the emotional blocks that they still carry from that life. The earlier Dai-Ko-Mio will assist to find and clear the emotional blocks that are limiting them in this timeframe.

The female Dai-Ko-Myo, named Modern Dai-Ko-Myo will resonate with the energies of current and recent timeframes, starting around 1980. The energy of the millennium is honoring the feminine, bringing back into balance the male and female within the earth and within each human form.

 The existence of the divine feminine has been denied for eons of time; this is aptly represented in the novel *The Da Vinci Code* by Dan Brown. In this book, Brown uncovers the truth about the traditions of the divine goddess and how the Vatican began a campaign to eradicate pagan religions and convert the masses to Christianity. Brown calls it a smear campaign against the pagan god and goddess, recasting their divine symbols as evil. His research discovered how the symbols were degraded in an attempt to erase their meanings. The pointed hat of the wise crone became the symbol of a witch and Venus's pentacle became 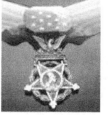 a sign of the devil. Brown reveals that even the government of the United States uses the pentacle as a symbol of war, as it is painted

on the fighter jets and hung on the shoulders of military generals. "So much for the goddess of love and beauty[1]," Brown says.

That said, this is not a time to dishonor the male and elevate the feminine; that would once again create imbalance. This is a time to blend and balance the two. This is why the Light Internal system of Reiki teaches all the Dai-Ko-Mio symbols which have been gifted to Reiki master teachers since Usui began his practice. Some masters have found that the original Usui master symbol feels grounded and energized, while the Modern Dai-Ko-Myo is softer, stronger and more calming. Both of these symbols have variations which are noted later in the text. Notice how each symbol resonates for you by using the inherent inner wisdom that is found within your heart. Then you will know when to use each symbol and on which client. Trust and know that your master energy will guide you.

Personal Master Symbols

Channeled by Reiki Master Students

Many Reiki practitioners have their own personal Reiki symbol. When this gift is mentioned some students immediately jot it down, saying they have sketched this all their lives and did not know it had purpose. Others find they can locate it by entering into meditation and asking for the symbol to appear.

The gift of this symbol may be revealed to you in a dream, during meditation or in another way. Watch for any metaphors which come to your attention. You may notice them appearing in your everyday activities, perhaps when you are observing nature or doodling on paper. When you have a desire to receive your symbol and are confident the symbol will appear, it will.

This will not be a symbol for healing unless you intuitively receive that it is. Mostly it will reflect your energy as a master. It can be placed on your business card or used as a logo. It can be invisibly embedded behind text that you are writing. This can be done as a whitewash in a word processing program such as Microsoft Word. You can place it in a document as an image and then adjust the transparency until it fades away.

---

[1] Dan Brown. *The Da Vinci Code, 49*

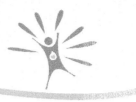

The following images were channeled by masters I was blessed to train. Some of the artists said this was an image they have been drawing for years, some since their youth. Others were able to draw it immediately in class and others came back with their symbol the next week. The fact is, they all found their personal symbol and so can you.

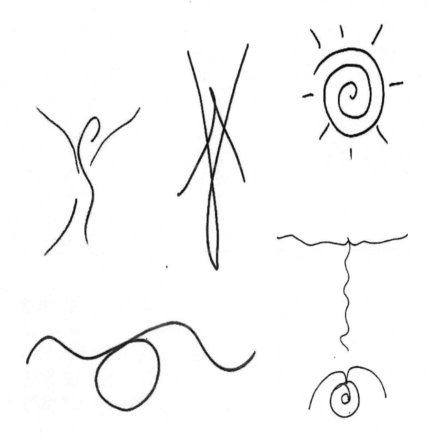

Personal master symbols channeled by
Reiki master students

Usui Dai-Ko-Mio

Original Traditional Symbol
   (dye coe me oh)

Translation: Great Illuming Light

   Dia   Big

   Ko   Light

   Mio   Shining

- Turns on Reiki master energy.

- The first traditional Usui master symbol.

- Originated in the early 1900s.

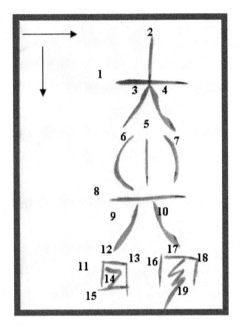

1.   This traditional symbol fits the energy of the early 1900s at the time Reiki was originally channeled by Mikao Usui.

2.   All variations of Dai-Ko-Mio's have equal power.

3.   Begin a healing treatment by drawing the master symbol.

4.   The master symbol encompasses all the Reiki symbols, so it can be used solely, as it pulls in the qualities of all the Reiki symbols, eliminating the need to draw each individually.

When learning a new symbol, it is helpful to imagine within the form a figure which is familiar to you. When a picture is placed along with the lines, the memory improves. This symbol can be seen as a stick man standing over another stick man. The second one has parentheses at the top part of his body. There are boxes at the bottom of his feet; one

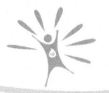

with a lightning bolt and the other with a sideways "V". Begin by drawing the first horizontal line from left to right and follow the diagram from there. All lines will be drawn for left to right and from the top to the bottom.

The horizontal lines #1 and #8 perform a steadying force to balance the body. The second line will direct Reiki energy from the cosmos directly into the crown chakra of the master. Lines #3 and #4 embrace the heart and allow this light to flow down the arms and into the hands of the master and then to the client. There is a direct line of energy which connects the throat chakra to the heart; line #5 embodies this. This is a force which is unseen in the chakra system but can become enhanced with conscious intent. It allows the spoken word to express kindness and compassion when this straight line into the heart is recognized and activated through intent.

Lines #6 and #7 embrace the emotional center of the solar plexus and blaze love and empathy into this space for the issues which arise during a treatment. It also creates a wall of protection so the practitioner will not take on the disturbances of the client. During a self-treatment it will allow the sender to embody more self-love. Line #8 establishes equilibrium in the body.

Lines #9 and #10 support the master as they apply energy to the legs; thus giving the master the ability to physically move forward on their path of enlightenment. The box over the right foot is closed and holds the energy of Reiki in their body while the left box is open to anchor energy to the earth. It also allows the nurturing love of mother earth to enter and blend with the cosmic energy of Reiki. This two-way flow greatly increases the healing attributes of the master. Now it is time to release the intellectual aspect of the symbol and embrace it.

In order to fully step into Dai-Ko-Mio imagine drawing it large enough so it may completely cover your entire body, stepping into it, as you will. This can be done in three ways.
1. Draw the symbol as tall as your form in front of you and then move into it.
2. Touch your body as you draw the symbol from your head to your toes.
3. Use your inner vision to place the symbol on your body.

Try each way and see which one brings forth the most sensations. It is not always necessary to create the symbol in this way, unless you care to; this is just an exercise to physically get in touch with the symbol. The master symbol will be drawn at the beginning of a treatment so the highest form of Reiki will be channeled. The other symbols may be drawn next if you choose. Illustrations of their order will follow.

Embodying the Traditional Usui Master Symbol

Becoming the embodiment of each symbol that is drawn is the practice of a master. This can be accomplished by imagining the symbol over the body instead of, or in addition to, drawing the symbol.

1. The Usui Dai-Ko-Mio can be seen with the first line drawn across the shoulders.

2. The second line comes down into the crown, which downloads Universal life force from the cosmos.

3. Lines #3 and #4 embrace each side of the heart.

4. Line #5 connects the heart to the throat, representing the voice of kindness and compassion.

5. Lines #6 and #7 hold peace around the emotional center of the solar plexus.

6. Line #8 stabilizes the body along the hip line.

7. Lines #9 and #10 steady the legs, encouraging the master to move forward on their path.

8. The box over the right foot is closed to encase the cosmic energy within the master's body, while the left foot is an open channel to the earth's light.

9. The left box, being open, allows for the transfer of cosmic light to flow into the earth, while mother earth sends her nurturing love up into the master's body.

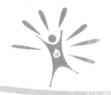

Symbols to use Before a Treatment

Before the start of a treatment draw all four traditional symbols, Cho-Ku-Rei, Dai-Ko-Mio, Sei-He-Ki, and Hon-Sha-Ze-Sho-Nen. Complete the process with Cho-Ku-Rei. The master symbol encompasses all of the symbols so drawing Dai-Ko-Myo alone will include the energy of the other traditional symbols. There are times I find drawing Dai-Ko-Mio is sufficient and other times I draw all the traditional symbols just for the enjoyment of drawing them. When I add the other symbols it helps me focus my attention on the attributes of those symbols and it really does not take that much longer to actively draw all four symbols. Cho-Ku-Rei or Fire Serpent can be added at the end to fully ground the process. The entire set of symbols may be drawn at the end of the treatment as well or just Cho-Ku-Rei or Fire Serpent.

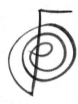

Cho-Ku-Rei
Channels the highest
power of Reiki
and seals the space.

Dai-o-Myo
Connects to the
master level of Reiki.

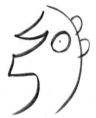

Sei-He-Ki
Floats issues up to
the surface and
opens new perspectives.

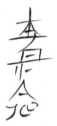

Hon-Sha-Ze-Sho-Nen
Directs Reiki to the core issue.

Cho-Ku-Rei
Seals the energy and grounds the process.

You may choose from any of the variations of the master symbols and use them at your discretion. They have been channeled from Reiki masters over the years and hold the integrity of the original master symbol. When they were first presented to me I was skeptical as to the power they held so I tested them out. I entered a state of deep meditation and asked my guides to show me if I should share these symbols. They said that because my path is one of an educator the answer was yes. I am here to present information to others, not to judge it. You have the opportunity to acquire your own guidance on how to use the symbols presented to you. Time is the best teacher. Play with the symbols and observe the results. Then make your own decision and know they cannot bring harm or be used incorrectly.

 Remember: Reiki is pure divine love and when one comes from the heart all things are possible.

It is suspected that Takata gave different master symbols in her attunements to various masters as she was intuitively guided. Since little of her attunement information has been recorded, this information is "hearsay" but nonetheless interesting to contemplate.

In traditional Reiki, when a master was attuned they were instructed as a master teacher as well. Nontraditional Reiki splits these classes into two so the master attunement does not give license for teaching. Because of the original way Reiki was taught the master teacher symbol is embedded in Dai-Ko-Mio and all of the subsequent variations. The master teacher symbol is a lightning bolt and can be seen at the end of the symbol in the boxes. In the following examples of various master symbols you will see the last variation is beginning to move towards the feminine energy, as the boxes have now turned to arches and the lightning bolt to an oval. The feminine progression is also found in the modern Dai-Ko-Myo which was channeled in the 1980s; you will notice it is very curvy reflecting female energy.

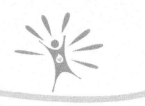

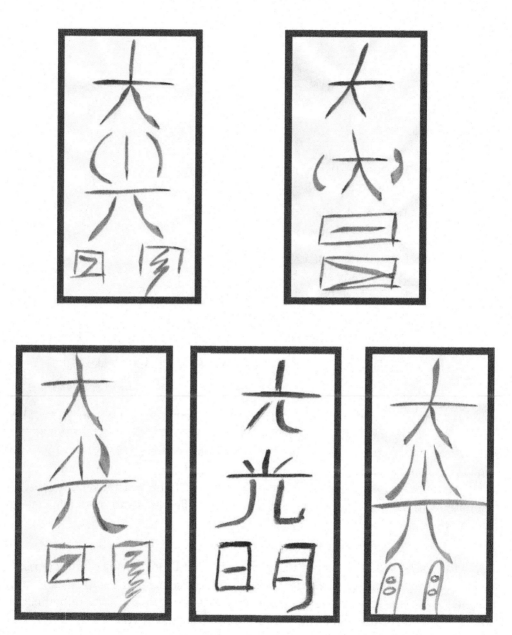

Variations of Dai Ku Myo, all have equal power

Nontraditional Symbol
    Channeled in 1980

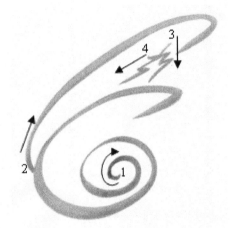

- Encourages the healing of the soul.

- Turns on the highest level of Reiki power.

- Encompasses all symbols and could be the only symbol to use if desired.

- Channeled to the earth and to Reiki practitioners in the 1980s.

- Swirl represents the unlimited power found in the galaxy.

    I first discovered this nontraditional symbol in *Essential Reiki* by Diane Stein. She describes it as "the most powerful healing energy on earth[2]". My master teacher instructed me through the use of Stein's book; therefore this is the first master symbol I applied. Stein does not say that she channeled this symbol and I cannot find reference to its origin. It appears very different from any of the traditional master symbols yet it resonates with the new vibrations of mother earth, reflecting a more feminine energy through the curved lines.

    As the planet raises her vibration and we assist her by increasing our frequency by having constructive thoughts and deeds, it only makes sense that the Reiki master symbol will change as well. Some masters see the symbol as astral rose in color or metallic gold. Draw the symbol in your mind's eye and see what appears for you.

---

[2] Diane Stein. *Essential Reiki,* 156

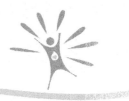

The master energy will travel rapidly from the healer's heart chakra to the heart chakra of the receiver and then into the soul. Before starting a treatment place your hand on your heart and on the heart of your client to physically honor this connection. When this soul connection is made it will not always be necessary to ask permission to give Reiki, for permission is granted on a deeper level than the physical. Even so, the soul can deny permission if it interferes with the free will of the client, so take time to make your request on this deep level.

Modern Dai-Ko-Myo carries the motion of the galaxy and the cosmos in its swirling activity. It begins in the center and is drawn outward reflecting the powerful force of a nebula from space or a tidal pool in the ocean. The second movement hooks onto the first and sends the energy out to gather up even more power. The lightning bolt is split into two forms, the first drawn vertical and the next horizontal. This split always bothered me. I found it difficult to draw this part of the symbol as it felt disconnected. Perhaps the purpose was to better hide the master teacher symbol by creating this division. As you choose your master symbol do not let yourself get confused over the numerous choices. It can be pretty easy to find the one which resonates with your energy; it almost pops out before your eyes.

 Remember: You are the master, not the symbol; the symbol is only a tool, do not give your power away to it.

When I found the next variation of the master symbol I ignored it for a few years. It seemed just like modern Dai-Ko-Myo but it was lying on its side. I was enlightened as to the use of this new Dai-Ko-Myo by another master teacher. He explained that this symbol is a chalice which holds the light of Reiki for the master and then some of this divine light is released into the client or out into the world. I liked the way the light of Reiki was held within the variation of this symbol and that the lightning bolt was left in its original form. This symbol has also been called Dumo.

Dumo

Also known as Dai-Ko-Myo
a nontraditional symbol

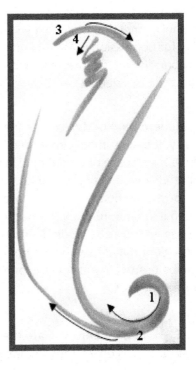

- Master symbol from Tibet.

- Stimulates the Kundalini.

- Aligns the upper spine.

- Seen as a chalice encompassing the body.

- Reflects the image of the Holy Grail.

This variation of Dai-Ko-Mio has the appearance of a chalice which holds the light and love of Reiki channeled into it. Besides connecting to the master Reiki light it also symbolizes the union of the mind and body and can pull all negativity out of the root chakra. It can be used to gently stimulate the Kundalini energy when the symbol is directed over the spine.

Kundalini energy is seen as a coiled serpent in the base chakra; once activated it will ignite a fire within each chakra to awaken them. All you need to do is ask for this activation and it will begin. The opening of the Kundalini can be a very intense experience for the body if it is done too quickly. Always ask for the energy to enter the client or yourself in a way that is harmonious to their lifestyle. That means it will not throw off their energy in the middle of an important business meeting or while in the process of

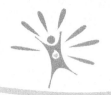

caring for children. It will slowly open the chakras during the night or when there is time to process the information which might arise.

Making this request will create a sacred space for the client to receive the healing without trauma to their body. If the process physically challenges their body and energy fields, remember that their guides can be directed to slow down and ease the process.

 Remember: There is no need to become enlightened all in one day. Enjoy the process.

When we are searching for our path, the Buddhist wisdom refers to the enjoyment of the journey and to non-attachment to the destination. As we go through life, the focus is often so intent on where we are heading that we forget the joys which we receive as we travel. Ask for your body to be balanced without excessive turmoil as you are raising your vibrations and transforming.

Embodying Dumo Master Symbol (Dai-Ko-Myo)

Dumo can be embodied by the following:

1. Visualize the swirl starting at any chakra below the heart.
2. As the left arm is raised, the left line moves up past the hand.
3. Raising the right arm allows the energy to move up, forming a vessel to hold the higher vibration of the high frequency of Reiki.
4. Imagine the curved line at the top, out in the distant cosmos.
5. The zigzag line directs the Universal life force energy into the crown.
6. Take a moment to feel the intensity of the master Reiki force entering your body as it fills the chalice. This holds healing energy and light for the master.
7. Master Reiki energy can now be channeled to a client, a location, a situation or yourself.

The symbol is easiest to draw in your mind's eye rather than directly on your body. You may fine tune the energy of this symbol by starting the base of the symbol at a particular chakra to intensify the energy there.

Example:

1. To open the heart, start the swirl over the chest.
2. To bring new perceptions and calm emotions, begin over the stomach.
3. To enhance creative thoughts, begin just below the navel.
4. For financial activity and support, begin at the base chakra.

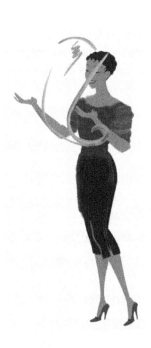

Dai-Ko-Myo begins at the solar plexus to balance the emotions.

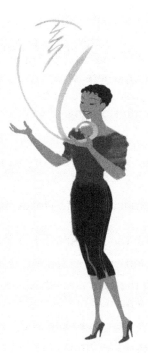

Dai-Ko-Myo starts at the chest to open the heart.

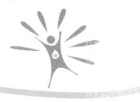

Remember: Now that you have been introduced to all the master symbols,
you may insert any of the master symbols in this series before and after you conduct a Reiki treatment.

1. The Cho-Ku-Rei symbol will open the path to Reiki and seal the space you are working in, with love.
2. The master symbol tells the Reiki guides that you are requesting the highest level of Reiki for this process.
3. Sei-He-Ki will allow prevalent issues to gently surface where they can be clearly seen by the client. In this way, the client can conceive why they are in the situation they are in, at the time, and accept their involvement in its creation.
4. Hon-Sha-Ze- Sho-Nen will carry the loving healing energy of Reiki to the original core issue to be healed, removing all barriers of time and space.
5. Cho-Ku-Rei at the end of the treatment grounds the process to the earth so the experience is anchored to earthly needs, desires and requirements.

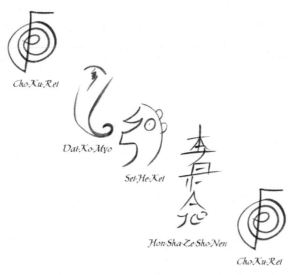

Cho-Ku-Rei

Dai-Ko-Myo

Sei-He-Kei

Hon-Sha-Ze-Sho-Nen

Cho-Ku-Rei

Before a treatment, draw all the traditional symbols and place the master symbol of your choice right after the first Cho-Ku-Rei

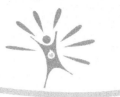

Chapter 3

Application of Master Symbols

The application of symbols may not always create the results required to completely clear an issue. That is when other techniques may be used along with the symbols. The Immune Energizer will strengthen the immune system by stimulating various acupuncture points. The entire process can take from ten to thirty minutes and is quite effective.

Crystals and stones are not only pretty to look at but have a vibration which can assist to raise the energy of Reiki, symbols, people and situations. They can be cleared, programmed, and used to continue the healing process after the treatment is completed. Their energy can also be applied when making flower and gemstone elixirs. By calling in master level frequencies, the master will enhance these liquids for their intended purpose.

As Reiki travels through the bodies of an individual its effects can be noticed in every facet of life. Sometimes this can feel overwhelming as energies are cleared quickly and may create an upheaval in the old life patterns. When the client understands how this clearing is beneficial and the stir up is only temporary, they relax and begin to accept the process as it flows at its own pace.

Dai-Ko-Myo Immune Energizer

Healing for self and others, from *Essential Reiki* by Diane Stein

There are times when a symbol is not enough to balance the body; in those instances the body may require a more physical approach. This can be achieved with acupuncture, massage or medical intervention. When using the Ran-Sei symbol, if you find it does not strengthen the immune system sufficiently, the following process can be applied. The master symbol will activate the acupressure points, thus joining the physical along with the esoteric.

The entire process will take about thirty minutes and can be shortened if you are so guided. The process involves rubbing a spot under the arm for 300 rotations and alternating between the arms for three rounds. Counting to 300 can be tedious so I suggest you watch the clock as three minutes will be about the time it takes for 300 rotations.

The acupressure point used for this process is a sensitive point located about three inches under the arm, a bit back from the center. Explore this area until the soreness is felt. For women this will be just at the bra line. The final step will anchor the energy into the body by tapping on the chest just below the breast bone at the thymus. As previously discussed, harmony is an integral part of the body's makeup. A healthy body works in harmony on all levels. By tapping on the thymus to the rhythm of a waltz beat, (hard, soft, soft; 1,2,3,) the body will pick up the beat. Think of music and balance.

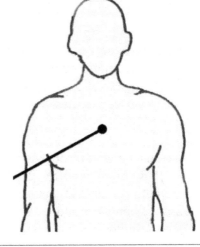

Thymus

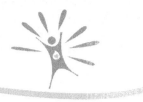

 Life Tool: Immune Energizer

The total time involved for the entire process as written is approximately 30 minutes. You may find this time can be lessened, so follow your inner guidance.

1.	Trace Dai-Ko-Myo over your heart and visualize it along with the other traditional Reiki symbols.
2.	Massage the sore spot under the arm using a clockwise motion.
3.	Massage the area for one minute while visualizing Dai-Ko-Myo.
4.	Continue massaging for 300 rotations, this is a period of 3 minutes; repeat on opposite side.
5.	Do this exercise on both sides under the arms for a series of three rounds equaling nine times, alternating back and forth between arms.
6.	Tap on the thymus of the client 20 times while visualizing Dia-Ko-Myo.
a.	Tapping can be done to the rhythm of a waltz beat: hard, soft, soft, hard, soft, soft.
b.	This will mimic music and will therefore encourage balance and harmony within the client's body.
c.	Complete with a full Reiki treatment

Clearing Crystals

Crystals vibrate to frequencies which attune with the earth and also our human form. You can easily locate the crystals which resonate with your current energy by familiarizing yourself with the qualities of the gems that are pleasing to your eye. Visit a rock and gem store in your area and start by picking the stones you find appealing and then reference their qualities in *Love is in the Earth* by Melody, or any other book which lists the attributes of stones. Very often the rock shops will have these books for reference behind their counters so request to see one.

It never fails, when I pick a stone which is appealing to me and look up its qualities, it holds within it just the energy I require that day. The joy of playing with stones in this way is that it can affirm your intuitive knowledge. When you find that the stones to which you are attracted are the ones that support you at that time, it will begin to strengthen and confirm your intuitive abilities. The confirmation shows that you can choose the proper tools, which in this case are crystals, without even knowing anything about a particular stone.

 Remember: The best way to increase your intuitive abilities is to make note of how many times a day you have an intuitive thought, and find it is later confirmed to be the right action.

Example: There could be a time when you are driving to an appointment and you decide to take a local road rather than the interstate. The local road takes you under the main highway and you find the interstate highway is backed up and the traffic is at a standstill. In that moment, make note that you followed your intuition and it was the correct decision. Keep track of these intuitive hits as the day goes on and you just might be surprised to find you are having numerous accurate intuitive thoughts all day long.

Programming Stones and Crystals

Stones can be a fun way to help children with problems they might incur. A stone tucked in their pocket can give them encouragement to speak up in class, diminish fear from a bully or alleviate nightmares. Find a time when you can invite the child to come to your home and pick out a stone from your collection. You may also bring your young friend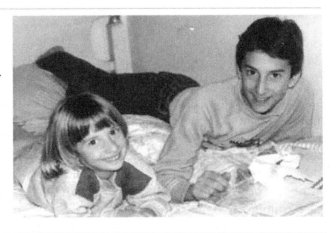

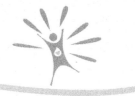

to your local rock shop and allow them to pick a stone which they like. Don't be surprised to find when you look at the attributes of this stone, that it is one which will help with the problem they are experiencing.

When children have nightmares, they have become stuck in the esoteric level of the psychic plane. When we are in our dream state, part of our essence moves out of the body and into the realms found in other dimensions. Some levels in the supernatural plane hold dark energies and we pass through all these levels before we land in the one where we rest, in our dream state. Adults have learned to pass through these levels in the psychic plane quickly and only get stuck in the dark places when they are overtired or extremely stressed. Children are not always experienced in knowing how to quickly pass through the negative realms, so they may become stuck and get frightened as they cross these levels. Parents may note their child will awaken with a bad dream early in the night or early in the morning. This is the time they first leave their body as they fall asleep and when they are reentering their body in the morning, thus passing through the negative psychic plane.

Children are often very aware of the esoteric world. They do not always mention what they see in this mysterious dimension because they think everyone else can see it. Therefore they feel no need to mention what to them, appears to be obvious. When you talk about these unspoken realms it supports their natural intuitive abilities and insures they will not lose this gift as they mature into a world which can invalidate it.

Before you council the child, draw in your Reiki light, use your master symbol and connect to the higher self of the child. Now you will have just the right words needed to put this child's heart at ease. Giving them a stone you have programmed will assist them in a quick ascent to the higher dimensions and a fast descent back into their bodies. The way you introduce this information to the child all depends on their age.

Example: Tell the child there is an angel who is by their side when they go to sleep. Have them pick a stone that reminds them of an angel, program it and tell them the angel lives in that stone. When they go to sleep put the stone under their pillow and imagine they are holding the hand of this angel. The angel will take them past the scary level and into the place where they can play in the light of the Universe.

Another child may be more comfortable with a super hero. You can use a figure of the super hero and tell them they will hold the hand of the hero as they fly out through the sky and into a place to play when they sleep. The hero is their protector and will take them around the scary places so there is nothing to fear. The hero is also there to hold their hand as they return to their body when they awaken. Program the stone or the super hero doll or the item they choose to hold, by using the "Life Tool" programming process listed below. Charge this object with the light, love and power of Reiki.

Any stone can be programmed to assist adults or children to achieve a desired result. Adults find the process helpful to relieve headaches, back pain, stress and the removal of addictions. The crystals or stones can be used not only to remove the negativity but to empower positive change as well. They can assist in clearing imbalances in the workplace, in one's personal life and in the dream state.

It can be fun to see what can be accomplished while sleeping, and lucid dreaming is an easy way to start. Lucid dreaming is when you are able to recognize you are dreaming and have the ability to interact within that dream. You may contact this state if you say to yourself right before you drift off to sleep, "I will remember my dreams and I can interact within my dreams." By giving yourself this conscious direction over a period of a few days, you can often attain the result. One stone which supports lucid dreaming is a green stone called serpentine. Hold it when you make your statement to interact with your dreams, and then put it near your bed, perhaps under your pillow.

In order to empower the stone beyond the attributes it already has and to customize it for the needs of yourself and others, program it with Reiki symbols and an affirmation.

- Cho-Ku-Rei will program the stone.
- Dai-Ko-Myo and Sei-He-Ki will assure it will be free from negativity and pain from the past.
- Dai-Ko-Myo alone will allow it to be self-clearing so continued clearing is not necessary.

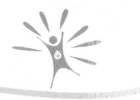

Prepare an affirmation to be absorbed into the stone, such as:

1.	This crystal consumes pain. This is great for migraine headaches or arthritis.
2.	This stone channels delta brain waves for a quick, deep and restorative sleep.
3.	This gem is activated to quickly and safely guide the holder to the higher realms during sleep. Use this when a child has nightmares.
4.	I will remember and interact with my dreams. This will assist an individual who would like to experience lucid dreaming.
5.	This stone holds magical powers and gives the owner strength, wisdom and protection. This can be given to a youngster who is threatened by a bully at school or if you suspect they are being abused.
6.	Stressful thoughts enter this stone and are transformed into peaceful vibrations which are sent back to its holder.
7.	Creative ideas are part of my everyday existence and I know how to apply them for my financial success.
8.	I find joy in everything I do and I find positive qualities in everyone I meet. This gives me confidence and inner peace.
9.	I am a desirable loving partner and I bring to me like kind, and until they enter my world I am patient, happy and confident.
10.	I breathe clean fresh air and relax with each deep breath I take. When a client desires to stop smoking this will help along with using the "Life Tool: Releasing Spirit Attachments, found in *Inner Gifts Uncovered, the Complete Reiki Second Degree Manual.*

1.	Hold the crystal or stone between your hands while channeling Reiki energy.
2.	Visualize all four symbols to clear, charge and program the stone.
3.	The clearing will release accumulated negativity and raise the vibration of the stone. Ask the gem to continue to be self-clearing.
4.	How it works:
	a. Visualize the Dai-Ko-Myo and the Sei-He-Ki encompassing the rock and the symbols will assist in removing previously absorbed adverse energy and pain.
	b. Send Cho-Ku-Rei as you program the stone for physical and emotional relief by using the affirmation of your choosing.
	c. When using the stone for healing, also add Hon-Sha-Ze-Sho-Nen.
	d. Use Dai-Ko-Myo and request that the stone will be self-clearing from now on.
	i. This will diminish the amount of clearing needed in the future.
	ii. For the quickest and best results, draw all four symbols over each crystal placement.

Flower and Gemstone Elixirs

Another way to implement healing is to apply the energy of nature through the use of elixirs and essences. Flower essences, as the name implies, carry the frequencies of flowers and other plants. The liquid in the bottles holds the life essence or matrix of the items that were infused into it. They can bring extended healing along with Reiki energy transfers. There are a few companies who make essences, but the ones I have worked

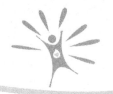

with are Bach and Perelandra. They are quite well known and respected. FES is another company but I have not tried their products: www.fesflowers.com

Bach flower remedies were created around 1930. They augment healing by using the power of Mother Nature. They not only resonate with flowers, but also with other plants and trees. A list of the 38 remedies and their qualities can be found at www.bachcentre.com/centre/remedies.htm

In the 1980s, Machaelle Small Wright, author of *Map, The Co-Creative White Brotherhood Medical Assistance Program*, created Perelandra flower essences, www.perelandra-ltd.com. Their series houses fifty-one essences made with roses, vegetables and what Wright calls soul rays. Both Bach and Perelandra raise their flowers and vegetables in a pure environment, free from pesticides and inharmonious vibrations. There are 38 Bach flower essences and 51 Perelandra flower essences.

The fastest way to find the correct essence for yourself or a client is with muscle testing or dowsing. Then dowse for the number of drops necessary and for how many days or weeks they will need to be taken. Testing with Perelandra is simple for they sell a set which contains all of their essences in 1/8 ounce bottles. They come in two small boxes and it does not take long to locate the correct essence.

To determine the essences required for yourself or a client, group the bottles together and with your pendulum, check to see which row holds the necessary bottle. You may also do this with a list of the names of the products you find on the web and then purchase only what is needed. There may be more than one required but do not use more than five because the body will not integrate more than five essences at one time.

Because these essences are vibrational you may be able to access their frequencies by writing their name on a piece of paper and have the intent to channel their qualities into your body. Follow the links above to review the products for each company and notice if you can sense a change. If not, purchase the items and download or ingest the product.

Example: I have found that the bottles I have purchased never need opening. I just place a bottle of essence on my chest, over my thymus and ask for their frequencies to be downloaded into my body. I see my body as a biological computer and treat it as such. I can feel the vibrations entering my body as their matrix blends and alters mine. I often feel an emotional charge when I use the essences in this way. In order to fully sense this activation, the bottles must be downloaded in a quiet environment when your mind is still.

You may increase the power and intention of any liquid used for healing by drawing Cho-Ku-Rei and Dai-Ko-Myo over a bottle of medicine, herbs, essences or homeopathic remedies. To save time, empower the bottles with the said symbols when the bottles are first opened. The intent will last until the product is consumed. Use this technique for yourself, family, clients or your animals.

Creating Flower and Gemstone Elixirs
_____

Even though these and other essences can be purchased at many health food stores, vitamin stores, and also on the web, you may find you have the ability to make an elixir yourself. The vibrations and results are subtle, but can be very effective. The process of creating an elixir is simple; the intended purpose for the essence holds a large majority of the power. So first be clear in your mind what you would like to accomplish with this essence and then locate gems, plants and other items from the earth which will support this desire. By searching on the web for the "vibrational values of flowers," you can find information on the qualities of various plants and then you will know which plant to use for a specific emotional or physical problem. Stones and crystals can be used in combination with plants for an essence and you can find the values of gems from one of the many reference books which are available on crystals and stones.

You will need a bowl to make the essence and also small bottles with eyedroppers which is where you will store the essence. Purify the containers you will be using by cleansing with soap, rinsing and then putting them into a boiling water bath. If you have ever canned fruits or vegetables, it is the same process. Fill the bowl with about ten ounces of pure water and place the cleansed bowl of water under the desired plant early in the morning or float the petals of the flower on top of the water. Say a prayer or affirmation which states your intent for this essence. Name the vibrational qualities of the plant you want for this mixture and ask them to enter the water and support the desire you have for its use.

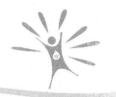

Write down your intent for the essence and then meditate on the process to attain guidance on how to proceed when using it. During your meditation recall the qualities of plants, crystals and stones you are infusing into the elixir and tune into their frequencies. Next connect to your sacral chakra to activate the creative part of yourself and affirm that there are no limits as to what you can manifest. To activate the intuitive information you received, send it up to your throat chakra so what you have created will be shared with others via your spoken word. This will empower you to share your newfound skill. If you keep your treasure silent, it will never expand.

Place the container in the sun for at least three hours or until the petals fade. You may check with your pendulum to determine the length of time needed for the infusion. After the allotted time recheck with your intuition or pendulum to make sure the process is complete.

Store the charged water in a dark bottle with an alcohol mixture. Start with ¾ purified water and ¼ alcohol; you may use brandy or a tasty liqueur. The liquor is used to preserve the essence, but vinegar can do the same if one has an aversion to alcohol. This will be the mother essence. To make the essence which is used, add only a few drops of the mother essence to a smaller eyedropper bottle of ¾ water and ¼ alcohol. Less is more when it comes to vibrational blends. Every time you dilute your essence, it gets stronger.

Example: Don't forget to add alcohol to the original mother blend. I forgot this step and years later when I looked at my essence there was a white mold over the water. Interestingly, this was the relationship essence I created and apparently I did not require it anymore; for when I discovered the mold I was packing up my possessions and moving to Tucson to be with my new husband. A detailed procedure on how to make an elixir can be found in *Healers Manual* by Ted Andrews.

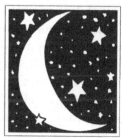

In 2000, I created a star essence to balance relationships and to create a sacred union between individuals, self and spirit, the cosmos and the earth, and all that is within life. I used the high energy of the stars, blended with the five elements of earth, fire, water, wood and air. Three days before a transforming planetary alignment, I received information from my higher self on the procedure I would use to make the elixir. I continued to access the information on the process for days. Planetary alignments happen on occasion and can be found on the web, but be cautious on the value you give this information for what is shared is not always constructive. For myself, I only focus on the positive alignments. One such activity happened on May 5th, 2000. It was called the Birth of The Age of Aquarius. That was the day I decided to make my essence.

I followed the guidance I received in meditation as well as the things that came to mind during the days which proceeded May 5th. As I started to prepare for the making of the essence I felt the presence of a council of four divine masters. To acknowledge them I placed four chairs in my yard near the pond. I felt this would honor them and make a connection to these great beings and be a reflection of their physical presence.

Beside the chairs I set a bowl filled with purified water, aligning specially chosen rocks around it. The first gem was angelite, a light blue stone used to open the heart; next was citrine, for balanced finances and finally a large quartz crystal, which held the original goddess energy of the planet.

I added to the mix all the elements found in the practice of Feng Shui. Feng Shui is the ancient Chinese practice to achieve harmony, balance and esthetic design. It is accomplished with placement and arrangement of articles in a space. The five elements used are water, earth, wood, metal and fire. I represented them all; the bowl of purified water rested on three copper rods, placed upon the ground near the pond, with a candle on a wooden base ready to be lit. I tuned in to my inner guidance and developed a ceremony to charge the essence.

On the night of May 5th, 2000, I began the ceremony to empower the essence. I sat by the water and lit a candle while meditating in the cool night air. I lay down and gazed at the stars above and asked for the power of the planetary alignment to infuse into the mixture. I intuited information about Soltar, the place of my soul's origin, and invited that divine frequency to infuse into the liquid. After thirty minutes I sensed the process was complete so I went to bed, leaving the blend to develop into a strong elixir.

I suddenly awoke at midnight with the compelling desire to retrieve the essence from the night sky. I walked outside and as I looked into the sky I found my intuition was correct. The clouds were moving in and about to cover the stars. I brought my brew into the house and placed it under my bed. For three days it continued to absorb frequencies

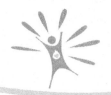

from the places I traveled during sleep. This became the necessary vibrations for the full development of the essence. I had never created an infused substance before so I had no model to draw from, yet the entire process felt right. When you make your elixir remember you cannot do it wrong. Allow your guidance to come from your heart and all will unfold in divine order.

Clients who have used the essence I created have found it assists in understanding and perceiving relationships in new and balanced ways.

Example: Joan wanted the essence to relieve tension between herself and her father. She was delighted to find that the essence did exactly what she wanted. Her intention added to the power already held within the essence. When a blend is created, know that strong intentions from the user can double its power.

There is no magic in the elixir; the force is within the individual. The elixir is a tool and can give assistance, but alone it would do nothing. When a tool is given to a client, make sure they understand their participation in the process. The tool will aid in reinforcing their constructive desires, but the power ultimately is within their own hearts. The Reiki master holds a sacred space to allow the client to step into their own self-healing. The way of a true master is in acknowledging the gifts which lie in others, thus empowering those who come near.

 Life Tool: Making a Flower and Gem Essence

1.	Create a strong intent for the qualities you desire to be in this essence.
2.	Cleanse a glass container by washing with detergent, rinsing it and then placing it in a boiling water bath for 15 minutes.
3.	Fill the container with 10 ounces of purified water and place it under the plant you wish to infuse early in the morning. You may also float the petals of the flower on top of the water.
4.	Place the container in the sun for at least three hours or the time you have intuited it requires.

5.	When the time is up, empty the contents into a dark bottle and add 2 ounces of alcohol or vinegar.
6.	This is the mother essence. Place a few drop of this essence into a smaller dark eyedropper bottle and add ¼ alcohol to ¾ purified water. This will be the remedy.
7.	A few drops of the remedy can be placed in a glass of water, under the tongue or on the wrist. It can also be placed on the paws of animals or a few drops put in their water.

 Remember: When applying an essence, less is more. The concentration of an essence will increase when just a small amount is used.

Healing Crisis

After a treatment the body is changing and adjusting so quickly it can experience discomfort for a brief period of time; it is rare, but still worth mentioning. During healing treatments, whether massage, body work or energy work, the client may move energies so fast that they may feel worse before they feel better. As the intensity of the energy increases, more blood will flow into the afflicted area, which may for a short time cause uneasiness. The increased circulation will move stagnant toxins quickly out of the body which could cause symptoms such as a headache, body aches, upset digestion, fatigue or emotional upheaval. This is called a healing crisis or cleanse and it will only last about 24 hours after the session.

 Remember: Reiki works with the highest essence of the client's being, therefore every experience is held in divine order.

The session is always guided by the higher self of the client and therefore will not open them to more than they can physically or emotionally handle at the time. If an issue

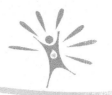

surfaces, whether physical, mental or emotional, then they have, on some level, asked for a new perception and all that comes with it, at this time. They are ready to move to the next level and clear the issues presented. As a Reiki master, you will be channeling the pure divine love of Reiki into all of their bodies, which will always soften their process. Love will radiate through the client as new perceptions are revealed, thus making their experience understood at a level deeper than previously seen and making it more palatable.

During the session the body is raised up to a higher frequency and this change will clean out what no longer vibrates in the body's new energetic field. This clearing could feel uncomfortable if it is not fully understood. Instruct your client to inform you of any dramatic changes they notice in the next few days. This will give you an opportunity to offer an explanation as to why they might be feeling distressed. In the case of colds, the lungs may need to release toxins; once these contaminants are let go, the body recovers quickly. Flu symptoms may intensify as the body expels virus and bacteria germs.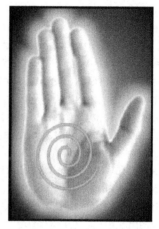

This type of cleansing or healing crisis can happen on an emotional level as well as the physical. When an emotional issue is approached with a treatment, the energy of Reiki will travel into all aspects of the client's life which are affected by the current disturbance. Reiki brings in a new awareness, a cleared perception and an awakened intuition. Within the new realization, every aspect connected to their dilemma will be touched: money problems, issues of rejection, relationships with their parents, or childhood patterns could surface.

This can be upsetting to the client because they desire to feel better immediately but there could be stones left unturned which need to be revealed and addressed. They may feel that the Reiki treatment has made their life more of a turmoil than it was before the session. This is where the knowledge of the master's personal experiences comes into play. The client is having a lesser form of the cleanse that happens after the intense vibrational shift from a Reiki attunement. By sharing some of your personal examples which occurred during your release in the attunement clearings with your levels of Reiki, you will help the client integrate and realize normalcy in their personal healing process. This will help the client better understand their personal development via a Reiki treatment.

The client is processing information at a rapid rate during an hour treatment and the vast knowledge you share with a client about their personal clearing process during that time can be overwhelming and may be forgotten by the client. Therefore, it is helpful to have printed information available for them such as a copy of the "Healing Crisis," "What is a Reiki Treatment" and information about specific chakras that are calling for attention. Some of these forms are located in *Inner Gifts Uncovered, the Complete Reiki Second Degree Manual*. A list of "Possible Changes During a Healing Crisis" will follow. Because clients are in a relaxed state, they may not remember everything that was presented at the time of the session. By seeing the information in printed form the client can read the data and assimilate the information in the privacy of their own home after they have integrated the new vibrational energy Reiki has given them.

Example: I received a call from a nurse who was concerned about her patients who were coming out of surgery. She observed they were already in a weakened state and she was concerned about adding more intensity to their healing process by administering Reiki. If she gave a Reiki treatment and the client went into a healing crisis, the nurse felt it could be fatal.

I reminded her that Reiki has a divine intelligence; it knows that the patient is in a state of recovery. Their higher self recognizes they do not have the energy to look at deep emotional issues during this time of recovery. The healing will be gentle, radiating love into the body and allowing the patient to access new perceptions at the appropriate time. The pure love of Reiki will be gentle and divinely guided.

When giving Reiki to others, be aware that it is out of the hands of the practitioner as to how the client will use the healing energy. We act as an advisor, who holds a sacred space for the client to step into and create their personal way to heal. As a guide, energetically we are showing them doors to greater awareness. They select which door to open and whether they have a desire to enter.

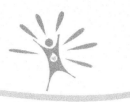

 Remember: When we heal at the deepest level, we heal through self-love.

The beauty of a Reiki treatment is that the receiver is blanketed with love and through that love they have more vital life force to experience self -ove, which will in turn become healing. If a person looks for alternative healing and their search reveals a Reiki practitioner, they are probably open to healing and processing issues at this deeper level.

Possible Changes During a Healing Crisis

1.	Reiki can, for a short time, intensify physical and emotional distress while healing.
	a. It can occur via colds, headaches, digestive disturbances or body aches.
	b. Minor emotional unrest, mental disarray or lack of focus may occur.
2.	These are indicators of deeper healing.
	a. Physical disorders may worsen for a short time, about 24 hours.
	b. Emotions may appear more agitated.
	c. Be aware that other aspects of life are also being cleared.
3.	Reiki works with the higher self and therefore will not bring to the surface any more than the individual is able to face.
4.	If the issue arises, then there is divine support to understand why they are being affected in this way.
5.	True healing starts when all imbalanced aspects of life are brought to the surface.
6.	For problems to fully heal, reorganization is required.
	a. All parts of life are connected; their associations will now be made clear.
	b. Energy could be distributed to areas other than where the

		symptoms lie.
7.		If one is working on clearing lack of money, deeper issues might be uncovered:
	a.	Handling rejection.
	b.	Imbalances and attitudes towards parents or authority figures.
	c.	Issues with responsibility.
	d.	Discipline, will power, listening to advice or letting go of ego.
8.		Thoughts, feelings and actions will be realigned.
9.		As these items are revealed, new perceptions will be perceived and understood.
10.		In this way, there will be a lasting effect of the treatment.

Even though most ailments are caused by deeply seated emotions, use caution in how you present this knowledge to your client. When sharing information about their physical state and the possible emotional involvement, alert them this is not to point blame; it is about awareness. You may guide your client to information found in the book *Feelings Buried Alive Never Die* by Carol Truman. This will allow them to discover the emotional components attached to their physical ailments. A list is found in the back of the book under "Probable Feelings Causing Ill-ness.[3]"

As the client locates their illness and reads down the list of feelings associated with an ailment, they have an opportunity to recognize the emotions they have struggled with over a period of time. By their own discovery, they will begin to see the tie between emotions and dis-ease. Presenting the book to them puts the client in charge for they are making the discoveries about the emotional tie to their dis-ease. This will also honor the divine aspect of their being which is all knowing and can become clear with the guidance held in the printed material. It is from the love that radiates through the practitioner that the client becomes cognizant of the issues at hand, without the client feeling judgment or blame.

The key to embodying Reiki is to trust the process, for both yourself and others. Know

---

[3] Karol K. Truman. *Feelings Buried Alive Never Die*, 226

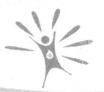

that what is happening, even if it is uncomfortable, is a stepping stone to a better place. If you or your clients are not getting what is desired, perhaps a time of rest is required. Divine order has intervened, making a place to coast until the next level is accessed. Let go of the expectation of how things *should be* and accept them as they are. This is the flow which follows a master and when the master understands this process he/she can guide others as they follow a similar path.

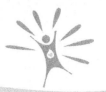

Chapter 4

_____

Reiki in Alternate Dimensions

_____

Intuitive work is accomplished in a place beyond our awareness of space and time. It is a familiar place to us for we travel there every night when we sleep but we are often not cognizant of the places we visit. In this chapter we will consciously enter these time/space continuums. When we understand how we play with time in our minds we can learn how to use the illusion of time to assist ourselves and others to clear past issues.

When we heal a disturbance held in our past it is required that we step out of the present and travel back in time to attain the necessary information to clear the old issue. We will be doing this with the support of divine beings of light that have the knowledge to protect our emotions as we uncover new concepts about these issues of the past. They can direct us to the place where we can remove the stress of old situations thus alleviating the pain. As we learn to process issues for ourselves in this way it will become easy to do the same for others.

As masters, we radiate an energy which draws to us people who are in need of help and require our assistance. Some of these beings who are attracted to our healing light do not exist on this physical plane; some are out-of-body spirits locked in a time continuum where they do not have the ability to transcend to a lighter place. Helping them is a simple process as we can easily aid them to move onto a path of growth and enlightenment. As always, there is assistance available on the other side so we do not need to do this alone. There are higher level beings you will become acquainted with in this chapter and you will find their presence very useful.

Everything we learn at this level is not always for the healing of others. Because of the path one has stepped onto as a master there are celestial beings who are here just to give personal assistance and raise the frequency of the master. With the use of crystals and sacred geometric movements, we can call in their help and our personal light can be enhanced. By the use of a "Crystal Energy Grid" divine assistance can be given to the master on a daily basis. Other grids may also be set up for clients and friends to help them on their healing path. It will only take a few moments a day to activate these grids, yet their force will be felt for a much longer period of time.

The Dimensions of Time and Space

When clearing any physical pain, emotional turmoil or mental stress, always ask for Reiki to go to the original issue. Then it will clear the current disturbance as well as similar ones which happened earlier in the client's life. When locating the original incident you will find it is often in a much earlier time, than the mind currently recalls. The reason Reiki can heal to the core is because we actually are traversing time and space. The concept of time is an illusion created by our lineal mind in this three-dimensional world. With Reiki, we traverse the dimension of time and become time travelers; even science will support the fact that this can be done.

Example: For many years scientists claimed no two objects could occupy the same space at the same time. Now scientists negate that premise because they have seen just the opposite in the String Theory. They have observed two objects in the same exact location at the same time, the variation being that the objects were residing in different dimensions. In the work we do, I see those dimensions as past, present and future. So we can be in the dimension of present time and change the emotions held

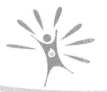

in the dimension of the past or bring supporting energy to the dimension in the future in a similar way that we give healing light as we lay our hands on someone who stands physically before us.

My friend Richard, a geophysicist, cautions me that I am giving a very basic explanation for a theory which is much more complex. Nonetheless, for our purposes this fundamental explanation will help to understand why we can make a difference in someone's life, even though we are clearing the pain from an incident that happened years or lifetimes ago.

Everything is happening at the same time, but we cannot see it because it is all occurring in other dimensions, which to our linear mind appears as opposing time frames. It is a blessing that we do not see all of these dimensions at once because to access all of this information could be a bit more than our thoughts could handle. To give this concept order, our mind has created time which does not really exist. Therefore, in our thoughts we slip in and out of these time dimensions and travel to the past and into the future while we occupy a space in present time. This is all done within the parameters of the mind.

Example: In 1985 the movie "Back to the Future," starring Michael J. Fox, depicted time travelers who traversed time but never left the physical place where they began their travels. They are shown in a car which can take them back in time. The car is on a street in a small town in front of a movie theater. When they ventured into the past they ended up on the same street only it was the old west but they were still in the same town. The same occurred when they went into the future. The theater was now shown as a dilapidated building. This fictitious story was reflecting the scientific theory that the dimension of time is what is being altered not the physical location. We too are time travelers; we assist others to enter into past memories in the effort to heal old hurts but we never leave our physical locations to do this.

Let's try out this time theory by seeing how quickly you can slip from one time dimension to another. Think of what you had for breakfast; sense the taste, temperature and texture. As you recalled the morning, did you see what you were eating or were you looking at the room? Did you see the newspaper you were reading and did you hear the sounds around you like music from the radio or the voices of others in the house? To make this recollection you just traversed time and entered into the past.

Now think about getting ready to retire for the evening. Recall your routine of brushing your teeth, washing your face or taking a shower; then sense the feeling of slipping under the covers. Are they at first cold? Does this feel good or is it uncomfortable until the sheets warm up? You have just moved into the time dimension of the future. You can now see how simple it is to use this same approach to traverse time and move into the past or future to help others clear issues.

This type of time travel has helped ease stress in times of war. There have been reports of people who have been held captive who kept their sanity by imagining they were playing golf or on a beach. This kept their mind away from the atrocities around them and made the time bearable.

Many young children who have been sexually abused have strong intuitive abilities because they also learned how to leave their bodies so they would not feel pain. One such child described going into a hole in the wall of her bedroom. This of course was only imagined but it kept her mind safe during her troubled time.

When a client protests that they are not visual and this type of guided imagery will not work for them give them this test. This will show them how visual they actually are. Ask them:
Think of the Statute of Liberty in New York City.
What does your mind's eye present to you?
What is your perspective of this icon?
Are you looking down at it or are you in front of it?
Is your visual perspective close or far away?
Did you see the water, the entire statute or just part of it?
Notice how you just moved through time and space, recalled images and in a sense, you were there.

People are more visual than they think and they will always see something when they have a guide to show them what to look for. This is a good way to show a client how time does not exist. One can travel by mind to locations and see them clearly, so they may also apply this technique to heal a past trauma because the mind does not know the difference between an imagined image and a real one.

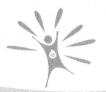

 Remember: Science has shown that the brain waves are exactly the same whether an image is pictured in the mind or actually seen.

When one goes to the original core issue, the effects can be erased or changed while in the process and the brain will believe it really happened in this new way. This is not only the power of positive thinking, but actually the way the brain works. Permanent change is not an activity of the conscious mind but of the subconscious mind. When Reiki is applied the client will drift into their subconscious mind where this everlasting change occurs.

Supporting and Healing the Inner Child

Almost every emotional issue has stemmed from an incident held in the past, often when we were much younger than we imagine. As we look back as an adult, what happened years ago may seem infinitesimal, but to a small child it was huge.

Example: I once heard a psychologist on a radio station mention that every childhood issue, on a rating scale from one to ten, has an intensity of the highest magnitude at a ten. As small children we rely on the adults in our lives to care, feed, love and nurture us. When this does not occur we are devastated. Just spend a few minutes walking around on your knees and observe how large the world appears when you are only three feet tall. It matters not whether the child was physically abused or ignored. For an adult, these childhood invalidations become life altering.

When a treatment is given with Reiki it has the ability to bring in a focus of love which was denied in some way to the child. The love felt will make most clients relax and allow healing of their old wounds. With love as a base, clients will begin to trust your guidance. Reiki will bring the client into the relaxed state of their subconscious mind so the treatment can relieve the stress associated with a traumatic event.

Remember: The subconscious mind rules the conscious mind. Enter the subconscious mind to permanently release the stress associated with any trauma.

When working with childhood issues, you will be guiding the adult or adolescent client to approach their younger child with the understanding and compassion they would hold for a child who was in the same situation now. By receiving Reiki and following guided imagery the client will gently float down into their subconscious mind. To open this aspect of their psyche, guide the client to open each chakra, being prudent to have them make note of any sensations they may be feeling. If they are not aware of any changes in their body, tell them to pretend to feel something. This will stimulate their imagination. You will find that usually by the time they get to the last chakra and often before, they will actually physically feel something in their body. Now they will be ready to use into their inner sight and help their lost child.

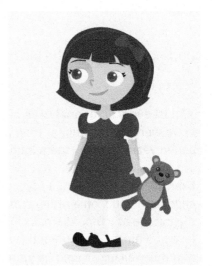

Once they are in this relaxed state you will start the process of Inner Child Healing. Request that they call in two beings for help; one is a guide to lead them down the correct path and the other, a divine light being, such as an angel. The client is creating this scenario so give them options from which to choose. This will assure them they are in control, have help, and are not alone. They will also be connecting to their higher self for added assistance.

It will empower the client if they can view their higher self and compare their radiance to the higher light beings they have called in. Have them look at their divine essence by asking what color is their higher self, for color is often the easiest visual to comprehend. If they do not see a color, ask what color would they like it to be and then pretend to see it. This is a way to prime the pump of their imagination and get them ready to view an occurrence during the Inner Child Healing process.

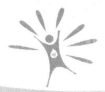

They will see how powerful they are when they compare their brilliance to the beings who were just invited in. If their light is dim it reflects a poor self-image. To adjust this imbalance, ask them to simply increase their light by imagining they are turning up a light in a room with a dimmer switch. This higher radiance will allow the client to work from the divine aspect of themselves, and when they see how simple it is to increase their light, it instills confidence.

As a practitioner, you can look at the episode they are re-experiencing as an observer and it is wise to direct them to do the same. There is no need to relive any pain of the past, though the process may stimulate emotions within them, but be assured, they will not be overwhelmed. When they are instructed to move to an old issue which requires healing sometimes the age the client first visits does not hold any trauma or concerns. Accept the information they share and after a few moments, invite them to go to a different age. The client may be entering an event which is harmonious just to trust the process and to get a sense of how it will work. This is an unconscious act. Once they feel confident with the procedure they will trust they can move into a place which requires healing.

Continue to be reminiscent of the divine assistance during the process especially when they need to comfort their inner child. They may hold this little one and ask what it needs. The client can then fulfill the request of their younger self. When the child does not express its needs, have your client think of what they would do if they saw a child today, in a similar situation. How would they talk to them to encourage them to share their feeling? Then have them do the same for this little one, their inner child. As a practitioner, you may practice the "Life Tool: Inner Child Healing" on yourself, to familiarize yourself with the procedure and as you process issues for yourself, you will become more adept to assist others. If possible allow a friend or fellow Reiki practitioner to guide you through this process.

 Remember: The divine is always in charge, so listen to the higher self of your client because it knows what the greatest need is and it will guide you and your client.

Once the child expresses its concerns, is appeased and relaxed, ask the child if they would like to go to a place where they are safe and loved. When they agree, bring the child back into the heart of yourself (in self treatments) or the heart of the client by seeing both the adult and the child, moving along a timeline into present time. One more step which will assure the issue is completely clear, is working with lights along the timeline.

Imagine a string of light bulbs which represent the image of a time sequence from the incident up to present time. Most of the bulbs are on but there are some which are not lit. The unlit bulbs represent a fragment of the earlier trauma which stays activated by memory; these memories can be cleared by the analogy of turning the bulb back on. This can be done by the small child.

Tell your client to give their little child the job of turning on the light bulbs. The children like to do this and they will find their own way to accomplish this task. Have them let you know when they have reached present time or if there is a light bulb which will not turn on. When this occurs ask them their age at this place on the timeline. To clear the situation, direct the client through the previous steps of Inner Child Healing. They will drop down and converse with this younger aspect of themselves. Once that incident is understood there will be two children that will move along the timeline adjusting the light bulbs. Each time a bulb will not go on, investigate the age and incident. Once cleared, allow the new child to join the group and help light up the bulbs. There are times when the incident does not need to be viewed. This is a time when the child only needs to be retrieved. They will continue this process until they reach present time. This actually becomes a delightful process as the client gathers the younger aspects of themselves and they all join together to reach a common goal.

Example: One gentleman shared his experience with me at the end of his process. As he picked up his little boys they jumped on a big yellow school bus which he drove. There were quite a few incidents to clear but most of the time the boys just climbed onto the bus as it became very full. The boys laughed, played and hung out the windows as they drove along the timeline; in fact they were quite rowdy. It became a fun experience and this was all done through the imagination of the client, not me, which empowered his process.

Another woman found as each girl joined the group, the older ones would help the younger ones. They would take turns going down and lighting the bulbs. After a time, the entire row of bulbs lit up like dominos falling down. It really surprised her how quick it was to clear the fragments of this old issue.

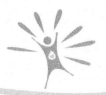

Once the child (or if there are more aspects of them, children,) reaches present time, guide the client to open their heart to make room for their inner child. So they may get a sense of this opening, have them take a deep breath and feel their ribs expand. Create a place for the little ones to be, and have the child design its own space. If there is more than one child they may want separate places; let them decide. It could be a beautiful bedroom full of toys, a dining room table where the entire family talks and the child has a voice, or perhaps an outside playground. Find what the youngsters want to make them feel welcome, and then let the client generate the request.

Remind the client to check in on this younger aspect of the self from time to time. Receiving this attention, the child will in turn enfold them with love. Ultimately this becomes an easy way to administer self-love, which we all need. All the Life Tools are advantageous as self-treatments for they clear the practitioner and create an excellent understanding of each process.

To locate the age of the inner child who needs assistance, begin by having the client lie on the massage table or sit quietly with eyes closed. Begin with the clear intent to find and assist their small, injured child. Start with a general Reiki treatment and follow with guided imagery of the Life Tool: Inner Child Healing. Affirm that they do not need to physically experience the trauma, but are entering the situation as an observer, to assist in any way they can, from the higher aspect of themselves. Once they are relaxed, ask the client to think of a number from one to ten. After they give you a number ask if it is days, months or years.

If the child who comes in at first is older, perhaps a teenager, after clearing the child at this age, if it seems appropriate at that time, ask the client to recall a younger child. The procedure is processing in its own way. Sometimes the client needs time to gently process a less stressful time in their youth before they can bring to mind their younger self who is more deeply injured.

Once they have the experience of observing their younger self in a pleasant situation, they can see they have the ability to access their inner sight and their adult is not being traumatized by calling in this little one. This will allow them to go to the core situation which can be healed. Trust all is in divine order and there are no mistakes. Just remember not to push a client to a place that they do not willingly want to recall, as they are always in charge of their healing process. They may need time to integrate the energies and perhaps on their next session they will go deeper. Honor the client's path as they present it to you.

When requesting the age the client wants to clear, always ask for a quick response so their left brain will not try to form the answer. This can be done by asking for the number and then snapping your fingers. They will often unconsciously respond right after they hear the snap. You will find they are often surprised at the time frame chosen because they can be very young. Tell them to imagine themselves at this age. Find out in this picture if they are inside or outside, alone or with another. Ask if there are voices, who is speaking and what is going on. Direct support to the child as the story unfolds, just as if this young child is in the room with you now, because they are.

 Remember: Time is only an illusion, set up by our linear mind. The imagination takes us across space and time so we actually are in the timeframe recalled.

Empower the client to know that they have the wisdom to give this small child guidance, protection and love. Allow the client to spend the necessary time with their inner child and when the child is appeased and relaxed, finish the process by bringing the child safely back into the recipient's heart, in the current timeframe.

The adult has retrieved the child and given them the love which was lost, but the child also has something of value for the adult. It can now remind the adult that they, too, are unconditionally loved. It is the job of the adult to check in on the child from time to time and shower it with love. The child will then remind the adult it is time to relax, slow down, play with reckless intent and enjoy life. Complete the session in silence, administering Reiki and allowing the client to energetically integrate the scenario.

 Life Tool: Inner Child Healing

1.	Place your hands on the client and begin transmitting Reiki. After about five minutes, begin to guide the client through the following process.
2.	Reassure the individual that there is no need to sense or experience the negative influence of an old trauma; they will be the observer over the

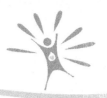

	situation, they have the wisdom of their adult and the assistance of higher level beings.
3.	Activate the client's inner sight by guiding them through the opening of each chakra in their body. Ask them what they are feeling and instruct them to give each chakra a color and temperature. If no sensation is felt, have them pretend they are sensing something.
4.	Request the presence of a guide and an angel or higher level being. Their presence will be noticed by the client's inner sight, a brush on their skin or another felt sensation.
5.	Have the client look at their higher self and observe its color, size and brightness.
6.	Compare their size and illumination to the beings that were just called in. If the client's light is lower, have them imagine turning up a dial until they reach the brightness of the higher level beings.
7.	Ask the client to move to the original incident which needs clearing. Ask them to think of a number from one to ten, this will designate the time.
8.	Question if this number corresponds to years, months, weeks or days.
9.	Direct the client to imagine themselves at that age. Their guide and angel are now by their side overlooking the situation.
10.	Ask whether they are inside or outside? Are they alone? Do they hear voices and whose are they? What is their emotion? Who is with them and what are they doing?
11.	Give support to the child as the story unfolds.
12.	If the client is silent for a few minutes question what is happening.
13.	Empower the client to know they have the wisdom to give this child guidance, protection or whatever they are in need of at this time.
14.	As the child recovers from the negative situation allow the client to take a moment to support their child and hold them in their arms.
15.	Once the child is consoled, ask the child if they would like to go to a place where they can play, where they are always loved and totally protected.
16.	Have them pick the child up and set them up onto a timeline which leads into present time.

17.	Show the child there are light bulbs to guide them back to present time but some may not be lit. Their job is to go down and turn the bulbs back on.
18.	Tell the child to let us know if a light will not go. Then find what age this is at on the time sequence and then guide them to clear the incident by following steps #9 to #17.
19.	Now both children are turning on the light bulbs.
20.	Tell the client, "Let me know if there is a bulb which will not go on or when you get to present time." Other children may join in the process; invite them to do so.
21.	Once complete allow the client, along with the youngster/s, to design a place in their heart for the child/children to be. Fill the area with whatever will make these little ones content and happy.
22.	The child's job is to remind the adult to slow down, relax, play and have fun. The adult's job is to remember to acknowledge the positive attributes of this little being and shower it with love.
23.	The adult and the child now have the ability to continually administer love to each other, which holds the healing effect of self-love.
24.	Finish the session in silence while administering Reiki.

Not only can you change a past incident in this way but healing can be sent to transform an emotion or old pattern. Use all three Reiki symbols and ask for Reiki to go to the core issue. Sit and think about the emotion or the old pattern and see what surfaces. A vision may appear from a life which is not during this life time; it could be a past life. Even if you are unsure about the possibility we have lived before, know the incidents you imagine could be from one of your ancestors. All of their history is locked in your DNA. Stay in the process until the original emotion subsides or a new perspective is reached.

Transition to the Light

The healing we administer for our loved ones on earth may also be given to ones who have passed on through death. After a soul has transitioned out of the body and into the

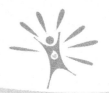

spirit realm, confusion may unfold within the soul. This can occur when death is sudden, as in an auto accident or heart attack. These are times when the soul does not have time to integrate what has happened. Don't be too anxious to give assistance too soon after their departure because they enter a resting period for three months and this time needs to be honored. This customary waiting period allows the soul to get in sync with their new surroundings. One can immediately ask for angels to enfold the deceased, but doing work to help their evolution to higher realms should be put on hold for a few months.

> **Example:** Before I understood the resting time period, I looked in on a recently passed soul. I found that she did not interact with me. In my mind's eye, she was very busy packing boxes and did not want to be disturbed. When checking in months later, I found a more relaxed soul. Her boxes were now on a truck and she waved goodbye as she rode off, with all her belongings.

Time does not exist on the other side; it is only physical beings that are impatient with the waiting period. The soul who has passed is not concerned with the time lapse so be at peace and know that when the time is right you may offer your assistance.

There is a lot of work to be done in the realm of the deceased for there are more spirits on the other side who need assistance than beings on this physical plane. The basics of Reiki are that it is channeled energy and does not drain the practitioner of their own vital life force. A Reiki master should be solid in this knowledge when working with disembodies beings and therefore have no reason to worry about spirits attaching to them while they are assisting the deceased. In fact, you may call in specific helpers from the other side where you need not become involved with the deceased spirit at all. The introduction of the passed spirit to these beings is often all that is needed.

Assistance from the Other Side

There are generally three types of beings who are well versed in the process of soul retrievals: angels, guides and helpers. After calling for assistance from these beings and introducing them to the deceased, the master may simply watch the process as an observer. This relieves the master of any responsibility or attachment to the results.

Angels are divine beings sent from source; they act as the fingers of God. Not everyone is comfortable calling in angels so use the term which suits your client by letting them name the divine being. Listen carefully to your client when they first come in for a session. Note the terminology they use and then choose similar words.

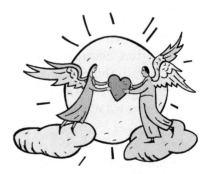

Guides can be specific in the assistance they give so always call for a guide who is familiar with the process required. When working with a client, if you don't call for a specific guide, you may just get one who is passing by who may not fulfill your purpose. A romantic guide, like cupid, would not serve a client if there was a need to release addictions. There is nothing to fear because when your intent is pure, the appropriate guide will almost always appear.

If you sense a spirit in your presence and are not sure of its intent you may always ask them to show you their light. If they do not illumine the space, ask them to leave. It is just like having a guest enter your home; if they are uninvited you would not let them in until they told you the purpose of their visit. From that point you decide if they are allowed to enter. It is the same when working with disembodied beings.

Helpers are designed to move the spirits who have passed out of the body to their next level of existence. They are very easy to get in touch with. When working with the deceased merely request a helper and one will appear; it is as simple as that. They are like a host at a restaurant. They greet the spirit and then bring them to the place they need to go and let someone else take care of the rest. Their job, like yours, is quite simple. It is all about introductions.

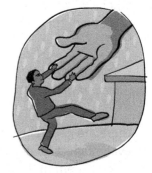

Souls on the other side often are not aware that they have passed, so they only see beings in physical form, ignoring the

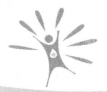

myriad of helpful spirits on the other side that are near them. The job of the master in this process is merely to introduce the deceased soul to a helpful presence on the other side that will be showing them their next step. In this way, the master is protected from any unbalanced contact with the deceased and allowing them their own experience.

Example: In the movie *The Sixth Sense*, the main character, played by Bruce Willis, had the audience convinced he was alive. He appeared to interact with the people in the story but by the end of the movie it was disclosed that he was indeed dead. The illusion portrayed is just how a spirit feels when stuck between the worlds. They will only try to connect with those who are in a physical body, usually because they have a message for them or they are just addicted to the energies of those in human form. By directing their attention to an out-of-body being, which could be an angel, guide or helper, you will help them become aware of their new surroundings and move on.

Buddhist tradition generally maintains that passing souls can not only hear and see, but that they also hold the faculty of smell. Once the spirit is released from the body, two of the five senses are lost, touch and taste, but the ability to sense aromas and to send fragrances still exists.

There is a Buddhist custom to prepare the favorite foods of the deceased and offer the bouquet of the meal up to them. This can be done for up to forty-nine days after their passing. This will comfort the disembodied spirit in their new realm as well as the people left on earth. By preparing this food the friends and family honor the deceased and are able to recall fond memories of their times together. This all makes sense to me for I am of Italian heritage and good food is always a happy part of our gatherings and instills sweet memories.

Example: During a session with a client, we were clearing some issues she had with her mother, who is still alive. When the session was about over my client noticed the scent of flowers and questioned if I could smell them as well. I did not but she realized it was a flower which her mother enjoyed. This touched the heart of my client and opened her to have compassion for her adopted mom even though her mom did not always reflect love to her as a child or even an adult. How interesting, that her mom on the physical plane appeared not to care about her, but was sending love though a fragrance from her spiritual body. Perhaps her mom really had a deep love for her but did not hold the capacity to give it to her when she is in her physical body. In her spirit body she could easily send her love. This is just a reminder that all is not as it seems and the divine in us is always acting.

I myself have experienced the perfume from Mary the mother of Jesus. It has the beautiful fragrance of a rose. I later discovered that is Mary's fragrance.

Use your imagination as a means of awakening your perception of what is happening on the other side. The intuitive process often follows an order. As you begin to pretend or fantasize a story in your mind's eye, within moments a vision will begin to manifest. Over the years we have been taught to ignore these intuitive thoughts so it could take a little practice to activate this part of our psyche once again, but with a little practice it can easily be done. As the tale unfolds, at some point a picture will arise which was not your creation; later this unsolicited image or gray area may be confirmed as truth when you share your experience with another who is familiar with the deceased.

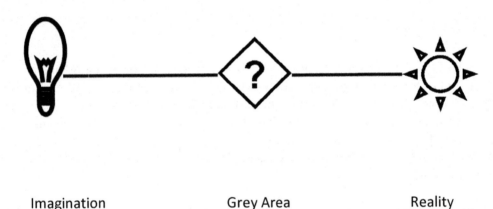

Imagination   Grey Area   Reality

Example: One of my students passed on from an automobile accident, so two weeks after her passing I felt it would be a good idea to check in and observe how she was doing. This was before I was aware of the three month rule. I saw her walking along a river, pacing back and forth, appearing agitated. I built a bridge of light to the other side but she would not walk onto to. It did not take long for a yellow dog to appear. It walked over the bridge and began to pace with her staying close by her side. I did not

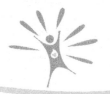

know whose dog this was, but it seemed to comfort Sue, so I closed the session, feeling that all was in order.

Later that week I spoke to our mutual friend Nancy and told her of the yellow dog who came to comfort Sue. Nancy had a dog that had just passed only a week before Sue's death. Nancy's dog was black, so I was confused as to why a yellow dog showed up. Nancy then told me that Sue had lost her dog a year ago and that Sue's dog was yellow. I was delighted to find Sue was being comforted by her own dog that was in the spirit realm. Once again I recognized a grey area, validated by the truth, which confirmed my intuitive abilities.

A simplistic theory on receiving intuitive guidance is to "fake it till you make it." I pretended to see Sue before she actually appeared in my mind's eye; I did not expect to see her pacing at the river or the yellow dog showing up. I started with my *imagination* and then I saw a scene I did not expect which was the *gray area* and when Nancy told me Sue owned a yellow dog, the *reality* of my vision was confirmed.

The act of pretending starts the flow of intuitive pictures. If no visions are seen, make them up; this feeds and stimulates the imagination and soon something will happen which was not expected. At that point, be an observer and let the information unfold. After the experience subsides, many times, confirmation will be presented to prove the truth in what was seen.

Example: A client named Mary came to me for a treatment on the tenth anniversary of her brother's death. She did not have a specific intent for her healing process, so I suggested that we look in on her brother and see if he needed any assistance. What transpired was very interesting and proves the "priming of the imagination" theory.

Mary and her husband were avid Harley Davidson motorcycle riders. As I started the process I kept hearing in my mind, bicycle. Certainly, I thought, I could not tell this biker her brother was out in the cosmos riding a bicycle, so I ignored the message. But the guidance persisted. I kept hearing bicycle in my thoughts, until I finally shared with her what I saw. I was careful in my approach to the subject, so I told her I sensed her brother was on a bike, knowing I meant bicycle and she would probably think in her head, motorcycle. Her answer to me was, "My brother did ride a bike, but it was not like ours, it was a bicycle." I was quite relieved to hear this and after receiving this confirmation I began to trust my visions, which opened my inner sight and revealed more of his story.

In the adventure before me, her brother was peeking out from behind a large rock and would not come out to be seen. I asked for assistance and a helper appeared with a bicycle. Her brother was very cautious with his new intruder, taking his time to interact. Eventually he came out from behind the rock to check out this new cool bike. The helper attempted to get him onto the bicycle, but trust was not yet established. It took a few minutes for her brother to release his apprehension. As he did, he moved out from behind the rock, mounted the bike and rode off with the helper. I knew then his soul was retrieved and he now had assistance to move onto his next level.

The last scene was a large rock wall which held no information for me. This time I trusted that the picture before me would reveal something to Mary, so I shared with her my outlook. Mary smiled and told me there was a place where she often sat with her brother and talked for hours. It was a rock wall at the ocean in California. Mary felt peace flow through her entire being because with this final piece of information she knew her brother was giving her the message that he was happy and at last free.

My intuitive eye began to open when I let go of my fear of being wrong and shared with my client what I was picking up. The *gray area* was the bicycle and her brother sitting on the rock. The *reality* was when Mary shared that her brother indeed rode a bike and that they often sat on a rock wall and talked.

It is easy to pick up intuitive information; the hard part is trusting that the visions perceived are correct. When receiving a message you need to call for the strength to share this inner sight with the client. Trust resides in the crown chakra, the connection to the divine. You can also put your attention on this chakra to gain access to information from the higher self of the client, then anchor this into your heart and share what you see. By focusing on the crown chakra you will have the confidence to express with assurance what is perceived, the power to speak this truth from your throat chakra and the support of your heart chakra so all will be spoken with compassion. This creates a very nice package.

With a little practice it becomes an easy process to connect a passing spirit to their appropriate location on the other side. When souls are too attached or addicted to

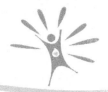

experiences on the physical side of consciousness, they can be reluctant to transition to the other side. The Life Tool: Transition to the Light, gives the practitioner and the spirit a path to follow which will assist the spirit to a new level of existence.

When someone loses a loved one, they often find it comforting to know someone can look in on the deceased to see if they are okay. Even if the individual does not understand the process involved and is not privy to metaphysical concepts, they often feel relieved to know there is help being given to their departed loved one. The bereaved is in a state of shock from their loss; and when they are greeted with an open heart, all things are possible and accepted. To fine tune your skills, practice visiting a being at their memorial service. See if the deceased is present. I find it rare that they are not. After all, this is a gathering of their closest friends and they are the honored guest, of course they would be there.

Example: During a funeral, the deceased gentleman was being honored by many groups that he had been involved with during his life. Many of them were military based and there was even a beautiful color guard ceremony. I saw him sitting in a chair watching the service and he appeared unaffected by all the rituals and the wonderful things people were saying about him. But when they played *Amazing Grace* he stood up in honor of his soul and I could feel the deep love he had for his divine self. It was a beautiful moment as it was a sense of love which I felt and it was difficult to put into words.

The mother of a friend had passed and at her service I saw above the altar two large wooden chairs. His mother walked in and sat down along with her husband who had gone on before her. They watched her entire service with a host of angels around them. There was a procession to the cemetery and they both followed us to the grounds and watched what was going on from the vantage point of a nearby tree. After all their friends had left her children stayed behind and shared their memories of their mom. When the stories ended and the children were ready to leave, their mom and their dad left the tree and ascended into the sky. I found it was comforting to the family when I shared my visions.

Life Tool: Transition to the Light

Use this process to assist those who have transitioned out of the physical body and are ready to move to a higher plane. It is best to wait three months after their passing before making contact. The process will alleviate fear and confusion for the deceased, gently familiarizing them with the new dimension they have entered.

1.	Envision a connection to the deceased. If you do not see them, make up a picture in your mind's eye. Draw the distant and master symbols.
2.	Introduce yourself and talk to them as you would with a friend or any stranger. Imagine they respond to you.
3.	Telepathically communicate with the deceased spirit to let them know there is no need to stay attached to the physical plane and you are here to help them.
4.	Dissolve any confusion they may have about their death while comforting and calming them. If their departure was sudden, they may need an explanation.
5.	Create an energetic bridge of light to the higher realms and see if they will walk over to it. Place on the bridge family members who have passed or deities.
6.	Other images may form which you did not create so follow the story presented, and be an observer in the process. Your next job is to introduce them to a being who abides in their new realm.
7.	If an image of a divine spirit or perhaps a family member appears, direct their attention to that being and make sure they look at it.
8.	You can also call in a helper and introduce the spirit to this being. Once you see the deceased interact with any of the beings on the other side, your job is complete. You may then step back and watch what unfolds.
9.	Stay with the soul until you sense they are at peace and have moved on.
10.	Dissolve your connection to them by drawing a Cho-Ku-Rei.

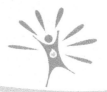

Crystal Energy Transfer Grid

The crystal energy transfer grid is a sacred space where guides will direct supporting energy specifically to the master whose photo is in its center. The angels and guides will be attending the grid to raise the vibration of the master. In the beginning, the master needs to be diligent by activating the grid often to build the energy and create a strong focus. As time goes by, the grid builds power on its own and does not need continued activation.

The grid is a powerful reservoir for setting intentions and a focus of light. Charge the grid every other day for a period of time, perhaps one to six months. Over time, you may forget to charge the grid; this is when the grid is clearly holding its own vibration and does not need repeated charging, so your attention is no longer drawn to it.

Example: One of my students used their inner sight and observed that one corner of my bookstore had a pillar of light. When they asked me what was in that corner I recalled this was the location of my Reiki grid. Interestingly enough this grid had not been physically charged for months, yet the light could be seen around it.

Placement of the grid is important, but not critical. You may place it on an altar you have already created or give it its own special place. It helps to place it where it will be undisturbed. I found out this is not always possible.

Example: I had an adventurous cat named Elliot, who loved to play. I set my grid on a trunk at the foot of my bed and after a few days, I noticed some of my stones on the floor. I did not give it much thought and placed them back in their appropriate places. The next day they were once again strewn across the floor. Still puzzled, I placed them back upon the grid, checked with my pendulum to make sure the energy was still in the stones and called it good. The next day I found Elliot whacking the stones, one by one, as he gleefully watched them fly. I checked the energy in the stones by dowsing and found their frequency was still high. I felt because he moved the stones in a playful, rather than a malicious way, the energy channeled into the stones was undisturbed.

Place your grid where it feels best, but know that the guides are able to work with crazy cats, unruly children, clumsy family members and gusty winds. When you hold a clear intent for your grid to be a focus to expand your light, your wish will be granted. My grid is in my bedroom because this is the place in my home where my personal energy radiates clearly without interference. The other parts of my home are used for teaching, treatments and entertainment, so they carry a vibration which is not directed solely to me. Because I meditate daily in this room, it has become my sacred space. Some find their grid emanates too much energy to sleep near, so construct your grid in a few different places until you locate its proper comfort zone.

The grid originally receives its power from the attention you give it when you set it up. Each of the eight crystals is empowered by the intention of the grid's creator. A photo of the subject is placed in the center of the grid with the subject's signature on the back along with four traditional Reiki symbols: Cho-Ku-Rei, Dai-Ko-Mio, Sei-He-Kei and Hon-Sha-Ze-Sho-Nen. There are six crystals that face towards the center of the photo, one crystal over the center of the picture and the eighth crystal will be held and used to empower the grid each day. The center crystal can be a stone shaped as a pyramid, a sphere, a double terminated crystal (a point on each end) or a favorite stone of the user's choosing.

Attuning the Stones for the Grid

Each crystal is charged with intention by silent direction. Enter a meditative state and hold each crystal, one at a time to empower them. Ask that it receives the full force of the Universal energy which will be flowing into it. The entire process of charging the crystals will take almost two hours, as you will be spending about ten minutes with each crystal to activate it for use in the grid.

When I set up my grid, I felt I would not need the full ten minutes with each crystal because of my extensive meditation practice. You could say there was a little ego there. The Universe had other ideas for the use of my time for the next hour or so. I did not set a timer but I was quite surprised that each time I closed my eyes and focused on a stone, when I felt my time with that stone was complete the time that had elapsed was ten minutes. It took three crystals before I realized I would be in this process much longer than I had anticipated. I must say, it was quite an enjoyable event as I felt the love from my guides who would be in charge of my grid.

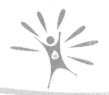

The energy brought forth into the grid begins with this meditation and as I found out myself, it would be wise to give the process its allotted time. The focus at the start will ensure a grid that will serve its user and be self-supporting in the future.

As you begin to set up your grid, anchor an affirmation into each stone. This statement will reflect your desires as a master and how you wish to share Reiki with the world. Each stone may have the same intent or different declarations may be used on each stone. You will know how the process will be for you as you proceed to charge each gem. Once the stone is charged, place it at the appropriate spot on your grid.

Initially Attuning the Grid Stones

Allow up to two hours to properly charge and empower all the crystals.

1.	Hold the first stone in your hand, close your eyes and take three deep breaths.
2.	Focus your attention on your guides and make your request.
	a. Attune this gem to assist in the growth and expansion of my inner light.
	b. May these crystals allow my inner gifts to be revealed.
	c. Make these gems a magnet to draw to me my transcendent healing abilities.
	d. Allow this crystal to have the ability to protect and bless my divine light.
3.	Remain silent until you are guided to open your eyes; this is usually ten minutes for each stone.
4.	Place this crystal on the grid.
5.	Continue the exercise for each of the eight stones.
6.	Let the last meditation be for gratitude to your guides, angels and the gift of Reiki.

Once the stones are in place you will activate the grid and continue to do so every other day. To activate the grid hold the master crystal in your dominant hand. Move the crystal in and out of the grid, counter clockwise, around the outside of the crystals which are set up in a circle. Follow the arrows on the diagram, remember to move counterclockwise and it does not matter where you start on the circle. Hold a positive affirmation in your thoughts or chant your desire out loud.

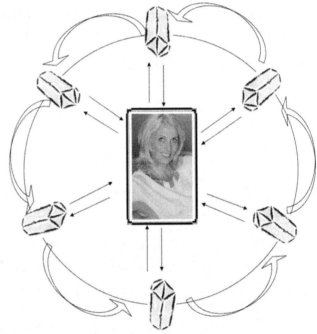

Activate the grid by holding the master crystal in your dominant hand and moving counterclockwise in and out around the outside of the circle.

The master crystal is used to empower the grid. Hold the master crystal in your hand during your daily meditation, prayer session or spiritual practice, to continually empower it. It will then be charged with your personal divine essence as it expands each day. It will also pick up a charge when you set it near your body when you are doing a Reiki self-treatment. Following your meditation or treatment, take the master crystal over to the grid and empower the grid while stating a positive intent for the day. Before you make your statement, connect with your divine essence, drop into your center and feel the shift. The following list contains a few suggestions; you may also construct your own affirmation, which is more in tune with your energies as a master.

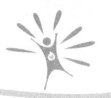

Affirmations for Daily Empowerment of the Grid

I ask this grid to be empowered so that I may assist myself and others towards transformation.	I ask beings of power equal to or greater than my own to continually assist my soul on all levels and dimensions of reality.
I ask for continual guidance, direction and clear intuition to keep me on my divine path.	I confirm that I love myself and that divine love pours into the focus of this grid, my home and all of my bodies: physical, mental, emotional and spiritual.

Charge the grid every other day to form the pattern which tells the grid guides that you are serious about your personal growth. They will then amp up the light pouring into the grid, which is going into the master whose photo is in the center. The grid will hold a charge for 48 hours before it needs to be recharged. Initially, consistent activation of the grid is important, but over time the grid will sustain a steady powerful focus on its own. The time spent charging the grid will form an integration of the master's inherent gifts and will continue for years to come.

The grid works on the inner realms through our subconscious mind. Also remember there is nothing outside of us that is not already within us. The guides, through the grid, will open the heart and inner knowledge of the master so that the master will come to terms with their own greatness. This understanding is beyond ego; it is a knowing which cannot be denied, invalidated or destroyed.

~ That which we seek is that which we are ~

The center crystal can be placed on the photo over the chakra of the master's choosing, to activate energy in that place.

Placement of the center crystal can be:	
1.	Over the chest will maintain an open heart as the master pours love to others while remaining open to receive love in their own heart as well.
2.	A crystal over the throat will insure that the words expressed will be divinely guided, truthful and compassionate.
3.	A crystal placed at the third eye will allow the guides to assist in increasing intuitive ability and accuracy.
4.	Placing the crystal on the solar plexus will calm the emotions and support a clear understanding of the feelings that arise.

A picture from head to toe will show all chakras of the body, but usually the focus will be on the heart, throat or third eye. Therefore a good photo of the upper body will be sufficient. The most difficult part can be finding the image which pleases the eye of the beholder. This is an opportunity to accept yourself just as you are, without judgment of being fat, thin, or old or using any of the negative self-talk which can plague our minds. On the back of the photo is drawn the images and names of the traditional Reiki symbols as well as the master's signature. This will bring in the energy of the master in present time rather than when the photo was taken.

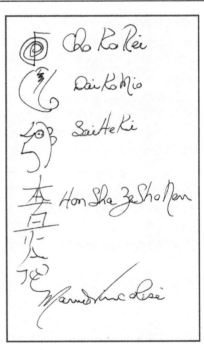

Backside of the photo for the grid

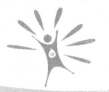

Choosing the Crystals

A traditional grid is made with clear quartz crystals to hold the purity of its form. My first grid was comprised of a few clear crystals, amethyst and citrine stones. The purple amethyst reflects the purple color of Reiki, the violet flame of love, and holds the highest vibration in the color spectrum, therefore represents the divine. I used the golden energy of the citrine crystal to activate continual financial abundance. You will of course follow your own guidance as to which stones to set in your grid but I did find when I made a grid of all clear quartz crystals I could feel a difference. The grid was more powerful and the energy felt clearer.

The crystals have a way of resonating with people and when you are shopping for them know they will call to you. While at a gem shop you might find there will be stones that will catch your eye, stand out and feel comfortable in your hand. They may be all clear or they may have color; you will know which ones to pick, for they are enticing you to come near as *they* pick *you.*

Once a stone is chosen, affirm your selection by referencing the qualities of the stone in a book written about crystals. *Love is in the Earth* by Melody holds a vast source of information about a myriad of stones. Surprisingly, the attributes of the stone which is picked often relate to pertinent activities happening in the field of the chooser. Remember these gems have attracted your attention and want to support your intentions and flood you with their healing qualities. All stones resonate to zodiac signs, numerology, and positive and negative physical attributes as well as emotional ones. Don't be surprised if the stone you picked just because you thought it was pretty holds the qualities which you are in need of at the time.

The empowerment or master crystal, which is held in the hand, can be very colorful. The following are some of my favorite stones for this purpose:

Rainbow Fluorite: dispels illusion and reveals truth; a stone of discernment and aptitude; brings order to chaos and helps with concentration.
Jade: helps to decipher dreams, connects to elders of the Mayan culture and opens access to the spiritual worlds.

Kyanite: will draw tranquility, has a calming effect, clears and activates the throat and third eye chakras and is a great attunement stone for spiritual ceremonies.

Lepidolite: activates the throat, heart, third-eye and intellect. It opens the crown, acts as a wonderful healing stone, helps with transition and restructuring old patterns.

Sodalite: brings direction and purpose, encourages self-esteem and is excellent for groups because it creates fellowship.

Rutilated Smokey Quartz: known to intensify the power of the quartz crystal. It is excellent for astral travel, insight and awareness. Communication with that beyond our physical realm can be attained by the using this stone for divination by scrying.

Scrying is the practice of looking into a translucent object or mirror and allowing images to appear, seemingly out of nowhere. The strings within the rutilated stone can reveal information through the shapes perceived.

Grid Setup

1.	Carefully choose eight crystals which resonate with your vibration.
2.	Create an altar for the grid in an area which will be undisturbed.
3.	Choose the strongest of the eight crystals for the master crystal.
4.	Place six crystals around a 12" diameter circle, points facing inward.
5.	The center crystal may be double terminated, a cluster, a pyramid or a sphere.
6.	Work with the arrangement until it feels right and then confirm the accuracy of your placement of the crystals with a pendulum.
7.	Select a picture of yourself and sign your name on the back along with the four traditional Reiki symbols and their names Cho-Ku-Rei, Dai-Ko-Mio, Sei-He-Kei and Hon-Sha-Ze-Sho-Nen.
8.	Charge each crystal individually for at least ten minutes, affirming that the crystal will activate powerful Reiki energy into the master's being and the world.
9.	Once the crystal is attuned, place it on the grid.

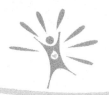

10.	Continue the process for each of the eight crystals.
11.	Activate the grid by using the instructions which follow.

 Life Tool: Daily Charging of the Grid

1.	Hold the master crystal in your dominant hand, drop into your center, then see and feel the energy entering your hand to charge the grid.
2.	Start anywhere on the circle and move counterclockwise in and out around the pie shapes while repeating a positive affirmation for the day.
3.	Meditate with the master crystal every other day and then charge the grid.
4.	If a time is missed, the grid will carry the energy into the next day.
5.	To send Reiki to another person, a project or goal:
a.	Use the same process as for yourself, but write symbols on the back of the client's picture or intended goal.
b.	Use a separate grid for each client and charge each crystal to hold the intent for the client.
c.	Reiki the written desire between your hands.
d.	Place photo or written intention into the Reiki grid.
e.	Charge their grid every other day.

Grids for Clients and Spiritual Coaching

So besides your personal grid you may construct separate grids for specific clients. For **healing**, create an individual grid for each client you choose and it will act as a continual stream of healing for the client. Place their photo (preferably) or their name in the center of the grid. Draw the four traditional Reiki symbols and their name on the back of the photo or paper. If possible, have the client sign the back of their photo. This will bring in their current energy even though the photo may not be recent. Set up their grid in the same way as yours: a powerful crystal in the center, six crystals at the edge of the circle pointing towards the center and a master crystal to hold in your hand to activate the energy every other day. Attune the eight stones for new perceptions to be accessed and to direct healing to the client. An affirmation such as "I am living in a perfect body" can be written and placed under their photo. The affirmation will change each week as the client clears issues and blocks. Charge their grid at least every 48 hours.

The grid can be used for spiritual, business or personal **coaching** to give the client guidance from their divine helpers and support their individual desires and goals. As a coach you will be giving directions according to what you have obtained from channeling information from their guides and higher self. Because a Reiki master is already proficient in connecting to the soul of a client, this process will be effortless.

The practitioner acts as a spiritual coach, using the grid to empower the energy with the guides, who are pouring their light into the client via the grid during the week. Thus the client will have the support from higher light beings which will then give them the ability to reach their desired goals. The master is then relieved from sending daily Reiki to the client as the guides are taking care of them. In this form, the grid becomes a very effective tool in assisting others to manifest their dreams.

The client will phone in on a weekly basis to attain assistance. To receive information unencumbered by the influence of the client, this process is usually performed at a distance rather than seeing the client in person. The coach will meditate with the grid an hour before the prescribed appointment. Because the grid is connected to the higher self of the individual whose picture is in the center, the advice will actually be coming from the client's highest source.

The session will begin with the client sharing what they would like to accomplish either personally or in the business arena. Each week they will call the coach and share what they were working on for that week and what differences they have observed. The coach will express what the guides are suggesting for continued growth towards the goal established in the first session; as goals are reached, new ones can be created.

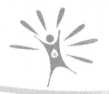

Affirmations for Client's Grid

During a counseling session with the client, determine the best approach for their continued growth. Create a positive statement for an affirmation which reflects their desires and goals. Each week the affirmation will change according to what they have accomplished. They will be clearing old patterns and gaining new perspectives on their current situation. The client becomes an active participant for they are also being given information, sometimes on a subconscious level, from their higher self. This comes from the energy which is channeled to them on a daily basis by their guides via the grid. Often the messages are accessed during sleep or while performing mindless work, e.g., driving, taking a shower, running and the like. Instruct the client to watch for these quiet messages for they can be brushed aside and ignored if the client is not made aware of how this process works.

Affirmations to empower the client's grid are attained through your intuition and knowledge of their current situation. The following are only suggestions and through counseling you will create the proper affirmation for your client.

I accept my body as perfect in every way: physically, mentally, emotionally and spiritually.	I am grateful for my gainful employment and enjoy going to work each day.	Every day I am building new, healthy cells and I feel stronger and stronger.
I love myself by taking care of myself in every way: physically, mentally, emotionally and spiritually.	I love the way I look, feel and present myself to others.	I enjoy moving my body through exercise or walking, and healthy foods taste the best.

Life Tool: Grid for a Client or Goal

This is a separate grid from the master's grid made to specifically channel energy to a client from their guides. It may also be used to enhance a project or goal.

1.	Use the same set-up process for the crystals as for your grid, but have the photo of the client in the center with their intended goal.
2.	Instruct client to sign their name on the back of their photo to bring in their current vibration.
3.	Tell the client to watch for intuitive guidance they will be receiving from their guides and higher self.
4.	Charge each crystal to hold the intent for the client using the affirmations previously given or ones you have personally created.
5.	As the weeks go on, hold their new weekly goals and their photo between your hands and send Reiki into them before setting them onto the grid.
6.	Charge their grid every 48 hours and be aware that their guides are assisting them on a daily basis via this grid.

If you enjoy using this crystal grid, there are abundant crystal exercises in *Love is in the Earth: Laying-on-of-Stones* by Melody. Many of the exercises given use numerous crystals; you may find the process will work the same when you create the patterns with fewer stones. You can be the judge.

Crystals sometimes require cleansing because of their vibrational qualities and they can be influenced by personalities and situations around them. Therefore it may be prudent to cleanse your stones before you use them for another project. Clear the crystals when they are first purchased and after removing them from a client's grid. The cleansing process can be whatever you desire; quick or ceremonial. Here are a few suggestions:

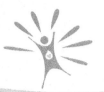

 Life Tool: Clearing Crystals

Crystals and stones may also be cleared in the following ways:

1.	Place the items in full sunlight from sun up to sun down.
2.	Cover them in sea salt and let them sit overnight.
3.	Rinse in cold water or place in a mesh bag and allow them to be rinsed in a clear mountain stream.
4.	Set under the light of the silvery moon, which works best in a full moon.
5.	Draw the Reiki symbols of Dai-Ko-Myo and Sei-He-Ki over the gems.
6.	Simply use your power as a master and request for the crystals to be cleared.
7.	Check with a pendulum to see when the process is complete for any of the above procedures.

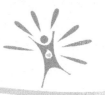

Chapter 5

Meditation

Reiki has a meditative quality of its own but you will find that when you start a practice of quiet contemplation it will increase your healing skills and intuition. When meditation is done on a regular basis, its vibration will begin to build, helping to lower blood pressure, balance brain activity along with enhancing creative and inspirational thoughts. Every time one takes time to meditate, the frequency around the individual is raised. That expansion stays in the location where one last meditated, which is why it is wise to meditate at the same place and the same time each day. The location will then become a focal point for quick relaxation of the body and stillness of the mind. When a day is skipped, the meditative energies are still being released by the individual's angels, guides and higher self, for use the next day. When a person makes an attempt to hold an internal peaceful state, there are a myriad of light beings that will assist them in accomplishing this goal. This will then make the process much easier for the eager student. If you have already established a regular practice of meditation then you will find as you move up on the levels of Reiki that your meditations will deepen.

Because our homes are not quiet sanctuaries and are used for multiple purposes, it can be helpful to add a physical focus to reflect a peaceful state. Light a candle, burn incense, focus on a deity, apply some aromatherapy and/or play soft music. If so desired, a simple altar can be designed with a scarf, the statue of a divine being, crystals or stones and the brilliance of a flame.

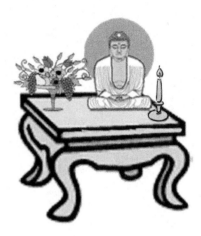

Meditation Altar

The best time to meditate is when the stomach is empty as the crown chakra resonates higher when there has been even a slight fast. The body uses tremendous energy to digest food and the focus will be directed to the lower chakras for this purpose; therefore try not to meditate after a meal. The times during the day which would be most advantageous are upon awakening in the morning, after the work day just before dinner or at bed time but not when you are extremely tired.

Much will be accomplished in only twenty minutes. When starting to practice, if it is too difficult to remain still for that long, begin with a five minute meditation and increase the time by one minute each day. Set a timer so the mind will relax and not be concerned with the expanded moments. It does not take long to become accustomed to this way of relaxing and soon you will find that the twenty minutes will pass quickly.

In the stillness of the morning hours, the higher self, through the subconscious mind, communicates with us. Guided messages, creative ideas and intuitive answers enter our thoughts just before dawn. When you awaken in the early morning hours it may not be insomnia; it could be your higher self trying to get your attention. Instead of tossing and

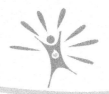

turning, tune to the higher aspect of your spirit and listen. Keep pen and paper on the night stand for jotting down flashes of inspiration. There is actually a Buddhist practice of awakening at three am for meditation. You are the best judge of when and how to meditate so try it at different times and alternate ways.

~ Great things come in the whisper of the morning ~
Rumi

Meditating with Reiki symbols or a goal, by imagining them in the mind's eye, will empower the value held in each image. The symbols will be activated by the divine to work for the highest good of the one who contemplates them. Sitting in a quiet state has its advantages, but with a clear intent for the outcome, the process will become much stronger. Be precise about what you desire to accomplish and have a distinct picture in your mind. This facsimile of the desire should be in full motion, already accomplished, now being enjoyed with immense gratitude. This moves one beyond the asking, past the work required to make it happen and into the grace of receiving this gift.

Before you begin your meditation, as much as possible, make sure you will not be disturbed. Inform family members or roommates of the intended quiet period you have selected. Turn off the phones, including the cell phone. It is amazing how the mind can be brought back to deadlines and stress with the tone of the phone.

Clear and clean your meditation space and you will find your mind will settle and quickly become still. Clutter in the environment is clutter in the mind. Ever notice how difficult it is to stay on track in the office when your desk is in disarray? The same can be said for the meditation area.

Be comfortable and warm, but do not mimic bedtime by lying down. The feet can be elevated, the head slightly reclined and a light blanket may be placed over the body. It is not necessary to sit on the floor with legs folded in a yoga lotus position, unless this is comfortable for your body. In India the practice of sitting on the floor is common and the bodies of yogis have been trained to be still in this position for long periods of time. In Western civilization we have not stylized our bodies to accommodate this practice, so give yourself a break and listen to your body's needs and sit in a way that is comfortable for you.

The mind has constant chatter; do not think you will quiet it just by sitting still. Allow it time to clear and do not become stuck on images it presents to you during meditation. Instruct this active monkey mind you will look at the ideas it presents when you arise but for now, see your thoughts on a conveyor belt, moving through and out of your mind. Start your meditative practice slowly for perhaps only five or ten minutes, as the mere exercise of sitting quietly can be enough to accomplish your goal for now. Stillness in the mind is accomplished over time. Remember, it has taken yogis a life time to accomplish this feat of a quiet mind.

Silence your Mind

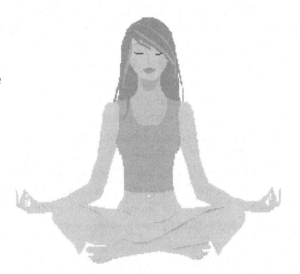

- Meditate in the same place at the same time each day
- Turn off all phones
- Get comfortable
- Sit, do not lie down
- Create a mood with music, candles or incense
- Be consistent

Let each meditation exercise be an example unto itself; do not compare one experience to the next. Just the act of sitting still has major benefits. Some days it will be easy to be quiet; other times the mind will race and there may be days when the body will not settle down at all. Give yourself a gold star for continuing the practice and do not judge the results. There is more being accomplished than what is seen by the eye.

 Remember: Meditation is a process, not a destination.

Each day that the mind is given the opportunity to be still, it will begin to integrate thoughts of the day, weeks and months. The benefits will be felt over a period of time.

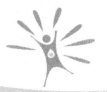

First it will be subtle and then more dramatic. By looking back over months rather than days, you will soon recognize the advantage.

If you fall asleep during meditation, know that this is what your body requires and that eventually the mind will stay semi-alert without sleeping. This is a new practice; give it time to develop without judgment and it will. It is repetition that will bring in the positive aspects of meditation. Some benefits noticed by people include lower blood pressure, clarity of mind and stress relief.

Alleviate compelling thoughts by writing them down during the meditative process. Opening your eyes to write a haunting thought will do less damage than allowing the idea to continue to press into the mind.

Be consistent. Fit this practice into the schedule at hand; the point is to lessen stress, not cause more by concerns about finding time to meditate. Some days are too filled with activities to stop and be still. Those are the days to be kind to yourself and do not let meditation be one more chore. This is a time for taking care of your inner being by creating self love and caring for yourself in this way. This can only be accomplished by letting go of demands and things you feel you are "supposed to do."

Honoring Each of the Four Bodies

When you are in quiet contemplation each of your four bodies will come into your attention to be cleared. They will each call to you in a different way. The physical body likes to be active but when it is allowed to sit still with no agenda, it will relax and allow the emotional body to open. This in turn will allow buried feelings to surface. When the emotions are given space to arise there is no need to run from them. The mental mind will attempt to make peace and give explanations as to why these feelings are here. Don't listen, it will only take you away from yourself and into the old patterns of denial or expectations.

This is a time to only observe what is happening. All that is needed to clear the emotional body is to be present with it. Each time you feel an explanation arising, know you have slipped into your mental body and it is trying to analyze the situation. You may merely make this observation and return back to the feelings in your emotional body. This is an activity which is occurring in present time. If the memory recalls an old situation or is projecting worry about a matter which has not happened yet then you are not in present time.

The mental body will never totally be silenced. It is there as a reminder as to what needs to be addressed next, but during the time you choose to meditate there is no agenda. The mind opens the doorway to understanding. The trick is to be aware of the pervasive flow of information and resist the idea to stop or control it. When the mind is allowed to upset the emotions is when the mind requires redirection. Usually, allowing the thoughts to flow freely without analyzing any of them will appease the mental body as well as the emotional body.

Within the spiritual body is solitude which is perhaps the most difficult to grasp of all, for it requires one to let go of all we hold near and dear. To step out into the unknown without a net, to walk an unfamiliar path and know that every deity you have ever called in is here at your disposal - that is the point where you truly let go and trust there is an assistant of the divine which stands at every turn.

 Life Tool: Guidelines for Meditation

1.	Meditate on an empty stomach.	
	a.	In the morning upon awakening.
	b.	Before retiring for the night.
	c.	After the end of the work day, before dinner.
2.	Meditate at the same time, in the same place every day.	
3.	Draw Cho-Ku-Rei symbols around your meditation area to clear, balance, seal and empower the area.	
4.	Clear away physical clutter to help clear the mind so it becomes still.	
5.	Build a special place in your home to meditate.	

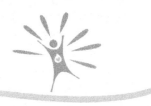

a.	Bring in stones, scarves, incense, flowers, music and/or candles.
b.	Make it your personal sacred space for these quiet moments.
6.	Twenty minutes of meditation is best.
a.	Set a timer for five minutes; increase the time for one minute each day.
b.	In two weeks it will be easy to meditate for a full twenty minutes.
7.	Make sure you will be undisturbed.
a.	Turn off the home and cell phones.
b.	Inform others in the house or office that you need your quiet time.
8.	Be comfortable but do not lie down.
a.	Cover up with a blanket because the body temperature usually drops during relaxation.
b.	Prop up your feet and slightly recline your head if this feels more comfortable.
9.	Do not rate each meditation as good or bad.
a.	Some days you will feel mentally active, other days physically restless.
b.	Just the act of sitting quietly has major benefits on its own.
10.	Keep a pencil and paper handy in case it is necessary to write down any incoming thoughts.
a.	This will alleviate thoughts from repeating in the mind.
b.	The mind will then have an opportunity to stay quiet.
11.	Even if you fall asleep, the benefits of meditation are still being received.
a.	Sleep is a signal the body requires rest.
b.	Honor what your body is telling you and respect its needs.
12.	Be consistent, even if you only give this practice a few minutes each day.
a.	It takes twenty-one days to create a new habit.
b.	Give yourself the gift of this quiet time and a new practice will begin to take hold.

Science has shown that the right and left sides of the brain function differently. The theory of the structure and functions of the mind refers to the two sides of the brain controlling two alternate "modes" of thinking. It also suggests that each of us prefers one style to the other. But if we learn to operate in both sides of the brain simultaneously we are more efficient, creative and relaxed. Certainly worth a try, wouldn't you say?

The right brain is our creative center, where we look at the entire picture. Our thoughts then can be very random, intuitive, holistic, subjective and synthesizing. The left side of the brain is our analytical side. It is logical, sequential, rational and objective. It focuses on the individual parts of a situation rather than seeing the whole picture. Productivity and clarity of situations come from a whole brain activity where both sides of the brain are used in conjunction with each other.

One way to accomplish whole brain thinking is through the breath. When we are breathing through both nostrils equally, we are integrating both sides of the brain. We do not usually breathe in this way. Stop for a moment and check your breath now; which nostril is dominant? The Life Tool Alternate Nostril Breathing, explained below, will quickly perform this act of whole brain thinking by balancing the breath. It can be practiced while sitting in traffic, though other drivers may look at you strangely, or at your desk or just before starting a meditation. When it is used before meditating it will still the thoughts in the mind, allowing for a peaceful contemplation.

It is important to use specifically your thumb and ring finger on your right hand for this exercise. The thumb has the acupressure meridian line/point for the lung. The ring finger has the acupressure meridian line/point for the respiratory, digestive, and urogenital systems. The urogenital system is the combination of the reproductive organs and the urinary system.

A cycle begins with closing the right nostril with the right thumb while exhaling out of the left nostril and then inhaling back through the left nostril. Then change fingers on the right hand and close the left nostril with the ring finger of the right hand while exhaling

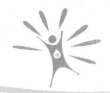

out the right nostril and then inhale through the right nostril. Followed by an exhalation out of the left nostril with the same finger sequence to complete the cycle.

Nine cycles are best and some doctors suggest practicing this four times a day to help with chronic illness, migraines, female problems (glandular) and chemical imbalances in the brain such as schizophrenia or multiple personalities. I have found it was very helpful with a student who suffered from panic and anxiety attacks. This young woman said that with just a few breaths her panic attack subsided. It is also a good Life Tool to use when disturbing issues arise, before bedtime, just before meditation or at any time that the mind is overactive and needs to be quickly calmed.

Benefits of Alternate Nostril Breathing
1. Whole brain integration.
2. Relieve panic or anxiety attacks.
3. Ease migraines.
4. Calm female problems.
5. Balance chemical imbalances in the brain.
6. Balance the right and left brain, creating whole brain integration.

Alternate Nostril Breathing

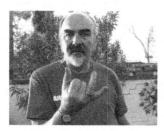   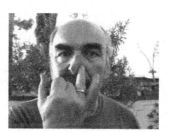   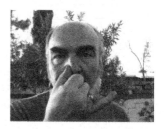

1.   2.   3.

1. Use your thumb and ring finger on your right hand.
2. Close off your left nostril with your ring finger.
3. Alternate to your right nostril and close it with your right thumb.

Life Tool: Alternate Nostril Breathing

Activating the right and left brain simultaneously

1.	Alternately close off each nostril with thumb and ring finger of right hand.
2.	Close the right nostril with the thumb of the right hand and exhale out the left nostril.
3.	Inhale through the left nostril.
4.	Change fingers and close the left nostril with the ring finger of the right hand and exhale out the right nostril.
5.	Inhale through the right nostril.
6.	Change fingers and hold the thumb against the right nostril while exhaling out the left nostril.
7.	This completes one cycle.
8.	Repeat this cycle eight more times.
9.	Four times a day for nine cycles is best; otherwise repeat the process twice a day, for ten cycles, once in the morning and once in the evening.
Advanced Method:	
1.	Follow the above process, except change the count.
2.	Exhale for twice as long as you inhale. This will clear toxins in the lungs.
3.	Another method is to exhale, hold the breath, inhale and hold the breath.
a.	The count will be the same for exhaling, inhaling and holding.
b.	This will increase lung capacity.

How to Reclaim Your Energy

Sometimes, no matter how hard you try, the mind will not let go of compelling thoughts from the day. This can make it difficult to have a stress-free evening or relaxing meditation. Guided imagery meditation is a way of using metaphors to quickly release the

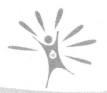

distress of these thoughts as it brings you back into the present moment. This exercise will eliminate stress and still repetitive thoughts, making it good to use before meditating as it will also help silence the mind. So when disturbing conversations replay in your mind know it is because you are not totally in present time. Part of your consciousness is at another location, going over the negative exchange. The energy must be reclaimed and brought back into the current timeframe to relieve the stress.

The following practice uses the image of a golden sun and a balloon to bring back your positive energy. The heat from the sun will melt away repetitive thoughts and emotions which are held in the body's energy field. The balloon will be seen over the head, back at the time when the incident occurred. The balloon fills with your pure energetic presence which is the energy you need to reclaim from that old conversation. This is required because part of your consciousness is still there arguing with someone or feeling invalidated.

This release can dispel pent up anger or judgment over situations. The whole process only takes only a few minutes to do, but its effects are felt for hours. Stress arises when the thoughts of the mind ignore the present moment and travel back into the past to rerun an old incident.

 Remember: The future is yet unknown and often does not appear as envisioned in the mind; therefore it is futile to worry about it.

To reclaim your divine essence start by recalling all the things that hold your attention about a previous disturbing situation. See the words that were said, written on yellow sticky notes and stuck on your body. You may also use the image of honey on your body. Imagine the emotions you hold are emanating from your body, out onto your skin in the form of honey or onto the yellow sticky notes. As they rise they are presented in a form which can be seen and therefore easier to release. Take a moment to access these thoughts, feelings and spoken words but do not dwell on them for they will soon be gone. Imagine your body is releasing the stress held from this confrontation as it lifts the memories you are holding in your muscles, organs, cells, blood, bones and chakras.

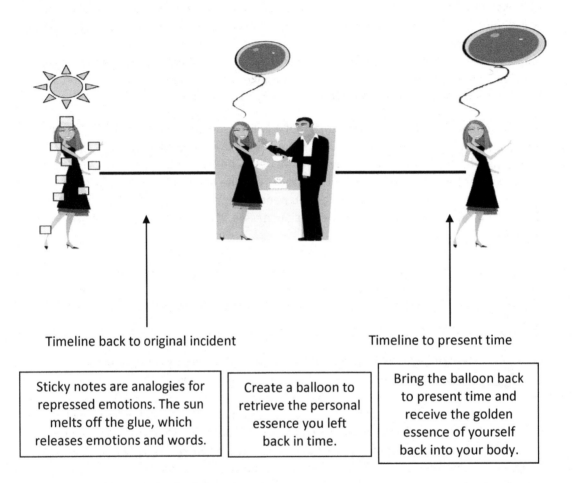

Timeline back to original incident   Timeline to present time

Sticky notes are analogies for repressed emotions. The sun melts off the glue, which releases emotions and words.	Create a balloon to retrieve the personal essence you left back in time.	Bring the balloon back to present time and receive the golden essence of yourself back into your body.

In your mind's eye create a golden sun above your head and allow yourself to feel its rays as it melts the honey or the glue of the notes, which then allows them to be cleared. The release of this paper or honey will let go of the thoughts and feelings you have held within. Notice your mind and emotions liberate; then move back along the time line to the old situation that you are processing.

See yourself with all the parties involved; place a balloon above your head and let your energy float up into the balloon. You are now reclaiming your essence. As it fills, the

balloon will become bigger and brighter. Then move the balloon back along the timeline to the present moment to complete the process. The balloon is now above your head, filled with the essence of you, the divine part you will now regain.

Imagine your crown chakra opening and allow the liquid golden essence of your divine self to flow from the balloon into the top of your head. Notice how this makes you feel. Can you sense which part of your body is filling with this light first? Are you more relaxed? Have the stressful thoughts cleared from your mind? Does the old story still have a charge? If it does, repeat the process and spend more time bringing the old thoughts and feelings to the surface onto the yellow sticky notes. There is no need to experience the emotions again, just sense they are moving out of your body onto the surface of your skin. Complete the process and notice how calm you feel.

    Life Tool: Reclaiming Your Essence

Now is the opportunity to release anger, stress and judgments held in an old event. If possible, the closer to the event this exercise is completed, the better. The process can be activated for present day situations or for those that have happened days, weeks and even years ago.

1.	Sit in a quiet place, in a comfortable position.	
2.	Close your eyes and take a few deep breaths.	
3.	Begin to feel your body relax as it becomes quiet.	
4.	Look at the old event and recall the discordant feelings, words and expressions.	
5.	Feel the negative thoughts and feelings begin to surface out onto your skin.	
6.	They take the form of sticky notes or honey all over the body.	
	a.	This brings buried issues to the surface to be cleared.
	b.	Each note holds words and emotions that were once locked in the mind and body; sense the release from your muscles, cells, organs, blood, bones, skin and chakras.
7.	Once all of the issues are brought to the surface, imagine a warm sun above	

	your head; sense its heat on your head as stressful thoughts melt into the light.
8.	Allow the sun to warm the glue or honey, letting the notes blow away or the honey drip off the body.
9.	Pretend to feel the heat flowing over your shoulders, across your chest, down past your torso, thighs, calves and finally off your feet, releasing distress into the earth.
10.	As the honey drains off or the notes blow away, so will the disturbing thoughts from the old situation.
11.	Stay in this warm sun until your body is totally clear and all the honey, which includes the judgment and stories that have been running in your head, has drained away.
12.	Move back in time to when the incident happened; create the sensation of movement by pretending to feel a breeze blowing through your hair.
13.	See yourself with all the parties involved.
14.	Place a balloon above your head.
15.	Imagine the balloon, like a vacuum, picking up your positive energy.
16.	The balloon will become large and bright; at that point it is time to reclaim your divine essence.
17.	Bring the balloon over your head in present time and let your liquid golden divine essence flow from the balloon into your crown chakra.
18.	As it enters, observe where you feel it in your body how the attachment to the incident has cleared. If there is still a charge, repeat the process.
19.	The second time, focus on bringing the deeply buried thoughts and feelings to the surface with the image of yellow sticky notes or honey.
20.	There is no need to relive the situation, this is only about clearing.

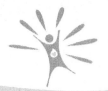

Heart Meditations

Meditations to open the heart can be beneficial on many levels. They will ease stress, activate new insights, dispel disbeliefs and increase healing abilities. Stress is created by the mind. It is a process wherein the thoughts travel out of the present time, into the past or the future, neither of which have value. The past has already happened and visiting old issues places judgment on decisions which were made by the parties involved which confuses and stresses the mind. The mind becomes perplexed because it is our innate presence to be loving and non-judgmental; when we do not work in this capacity we become puzzled. This reflects in stress, depression, low self-esteem and physical ailments. The future can change depending on so many factors that it is futile to waste time trying to analyze what will occur next.

~ I never think of the future. It comes soon enough. ~

Albert Einstein

When the mind is regularly given a time of silence, it will naturally begin to reestablish our birth right of self-love. It will also begin to reorganize thoughts which will make way for new insights and ideas. These quiet moments allow new light to shine on old situations, giving the ability to let go of previous beliefs which were not advantageous to a healthy loving life. Once a regular meditation habit is established, one which concentrates on the heart, healing will increase because the misdirected energy has a new more constructive course.

Every emotion has the base element of love: it is either present in another form or is showing the lack of it. Fear is the emotion which is merely the absence of love. When love is sent into the future then fear subsides. When the heart is open, new perceptions are activated and instilled. By accessing love on a regular basis, we release unnecessary fears often before we even become aware of them.

The Life Tool: Violet Light Activation will quickly open the heart and prepare the receiver to accept the love which is being sent from a myriad of sources, many unseen. The following exercises will show how the heart will be accessed, the body cleansed and from within those actions, love will emanate. Begin to open your intuition by contacting your five senses; sight, hearing, taste, smell and touch, as taught in previous Life Tools. This can be done by paying attention to your breath or imagining opening each chakra and creating a sensation in each one as you do.

To make the emotions of love tangible we will use the analogy of a tiny violet flame which will anchor in your heart. This flame represents the force which keeps the body at a temperature of 98.6, which in itself is an amazing feat. The violet flame will expand as it opens to ignite each chakra. Once the chakras are opened, the flame will spin around the body, creating a centrifugal force to clear out any disturbance which is held in the spiritual, mental, emotional or physical body. Give yourself time to experience the sensation this flame instills and once the physical and etheric bodies are clear you may extend this love to another person or physical place.

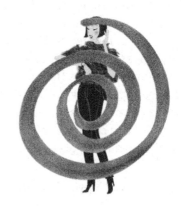

Start by stilling the movement of the flame and imagine extending this light of love to the heart of another person. Pretend to see them feeling this flame as you did, opening their chakras one at a time and removing all stress from their body. See them receiving this light with open arms and it will help to make it so. Make note of the time you were sending this energy to them and the next time you see or talk to them, inquire if they noticed a change in their emotions or activities during the time you were sending this energy. The change is subtle but apparent when one begins to open their eyes and look.

Example: A student in class sent her husband the violet flame. When she returned home she asked him what he did around 8:30 that night. He told her he did not know why but he turned off the TV and began to read a book. This is not a huge change but he stopped doing a mindless act of watching a program and became more mentally involved by reading. Another woman found that when she returned home from the class where she had learned and performed this Life Tool, her husband, who she sent the violet flame to, had a bath waiting for her with candles around it. It certainly appeared he received the message of love the flame sent.

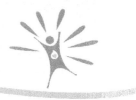

The beauty of love is that when it is given away it will expand rather than diminish. With this in mind you may also extend this balancing flame of love into your home, your office or a location of your choice. Secure the flame in one room or specific place in this area, such as a desk, and then allow it to build and expand through other rooms and floors. Every person in this local is touched by the love which radiates from this pure light. Pretend to see people responding positively to its presence. To affirm your actions, notice the next time you enter this place if the people are different than previously noted. Things may appear more organized, balanced or calm.

 Remember: The more love extended out the more love comes back in return.

The blessing of creating this image can be boundless miracles. Do not negate the power held in each and every thought we have. When a catastrophe is seen in the media a quick thought can send this healing love to transform the darkest of situations.

 Life Tool: Violet Light Activation

Here you will be able to fully contact the love which is stored in your heart. This tool will give the emotion of love a tangible form, which is a violet flame.

1.	Make sure all phones are turned off and sit in a comfortable position, in a quiet place.
2.	Close your eyes and take three deep cleansing breaths and let your shoulders drop to release any tension.
3.	Imagine relaxing into a pool of violet light which is comprised of pure love.
4.	In this light, create your personal sacred space.
	a. Open all five senses by giving your sacred place sight, smell, taste, sound and touch.
	b. Example:

i.	Remember the color of the grass; now imagine the color of your quiet sacred space.
ii.	Sense the air on your skin and note if it is warm or cool.
iii.	Imagine the taste of refreshing cool water from a clear mountain stream.
iv.	Hear a breeze blowing into your personal sacred space. Does it rustle through the trees or curtains?
v.	Therein locate a place to sit and feel the pine needles, sand, grass or fabric under your body.
5.	Allow the light around you to transform into a violet flame and place this image within your heart.
6.	Let the flame slowly expand as it soon encompasses your entire body, from head to toe.
a.	The tip moves up to the throat and down the base into your solar plexus. It soothes the spoken word while calming the emotions.
b.	The flame extends up to enlighten the third eye while descending into the sacral chakra to activate creativity. Notice any movement in your body.
c.	As it continues to move up, it opens the crown chakra at the top of the head, touching the divine while flowing down through the base chakra to anchor the physical body to the love of mother earth.
7.	How does this flame feel, is it cool or warm? Relax for a moment with this awareness.
8.	Rest in the love of the violet flame and focus on the opening it creates in your heart. If no sensation is felt, make one up.
9.	Activate the flame to clear the body by spinning the flame upwards around your ankles, calves, thighs, torso, neck and out the top of your head.
10.	Feel the flame spinning any cares, pain or stress out of your physical, mental, emotional and spiritual bodies.
11.	Slow down the spinning and still the flame.

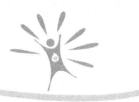

12.	Love expands in size when it is extended out to others, therefore, send this flame to someone.
13.	Imagine this gift of love anchored in their heart and then expanding through their body one chakra at a time. Follow steps #6 to #11.
14.	Extend this flame of love to a physical location, your home, office, a troubled country or any place of your choice.
15.	See this location enfolded with peace and love while imagining people in this place smiling as they receive its blessing. Begin in one room and then expand it to the adjoining rooms and floors.
16.	Allow the flame of love to blaze out the doors and windows. Stay within this imagery and see it build. Every person who steps upon the property is touched and transformed.
17.	When you are ready to end your meditation slowly come back into physical awareness by:
	a. Allowing the flame to diminish into a smaller flame.
	b. See it reduce in size but grow in intensity of color and emotion.
	c. It moves down through the crown and up from the base chakra at the tail bone.
	d. It continues to descend from the third eye and ascends through the sacral chakra at the navel.
	e. The diminishing continues through the throat and up into the solar plexus at the stomach.
	f. The flame now resides in the heart; notice how the color and sensation have changed. It could be brighter and more intense.
18.	Now that you have found this flame of love in your heart you may draw from it in times of need or stress.
19.	When you think of the flame it will immediately bring in the reminder of this peaceful state.
20.	Take a deep breath and open your eyes. Feel completely refreshed.

Another benefit of meditation is how it can open your awareness to better understand old situations and acquire new perceptions. When the body is given time to be still, the voice of the higher self has a chance to be heard. Besides the guided imagery meditations of the Life Tools, one may use sound to balance and calm the brain waves. One such technique is from the Monroe Institute, which is based in Virginia. Hemi-Sync is the technology they have developed which is a scientifically based method for synchronizing brain activity which provides access to specific and beneficial whole brain states of consciousness. This is accomplished by listening to CDs which have this special sound quietly embedded in the background of music or guided meditations.

I spent a week practicing how to still my mind by using their technology and it not only enhanced my meditations but gave me new insights while it opened my heart. During a meditation while using the Hemi-Sync CDs I presented a question to my higher self. I asked how I could increase the clarity of my third eye.

The visual which appeared in this mediation was an apparatus over my forehead at my third eye that looked like a telescope. As I contemplated this visual I found I could turn the telescope and receive advanced clarity within my mind. The effects of this meditation continued after I opened my eyes while I was listening to what others were sharing about their experiences from this process. When meditation is practiced regularly it is not uncommon to have manifestations and clear perceptions occur at unsolicited times during the days and weeks that follow. I must say, I did not expect what happened next.

Our trainer Penny Holms, the daughter of Bob Monroe, the founder of the Monroe Institute, began to tell us a story of when she was a child. Penny recalled a time when she was just acting out, being a typical eight year old. Her mom, Nancy Monroe, decided Penny needed a talking to. They both sat on the bed in Penny's room and Nancy made reference to a picture of Jesus that Penny had hanging over her bed. This picture did not console Penny for she never told her mom but Penny felt that her sister Laurie had everything better than she did. Even the pictures they had of Jesus hanging in their rooms reflected this. Penny expressed her disdain for this picture and commented that Laurie had a better one of Jesus. Her sister's picture had flowers and pretty colors while Penny's picture was dark and brown. Penny felt she had the short end of the stick once again.

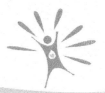

Nancy turned to Penny and said, "Do you see this picture of Jesus?" Penny was still not happy and recalled how she continued to feel this dark drab picture wass not up to par with Laurie's. Her mom continued, "What do you notice about it? Can you see there is no knob on the door?" Penny thought, but still did not get the full meaning. Nancy continued, "It can only be opened from the inside."

I was raised in a Christian household and this picture is very familiar to me, yet I never noticed the missing door knob. I remember it from my Sunday school class at church; Jesus is standing in front of a dark brown wood door and is knocking upon it. I never realized the true meaning of that picture until then. This new perception began to process through my entire body. I felt my vision of the telescope at my forehead and the opening of my inner sight was coming into manifestation.

I then realized the meaning this picture had for me. I had been searching for a loving relationship and did not realize why it had not manifested. Now I could see no one was going to enter my domain, which is my heart, until I pushed open the door; it must be accessed from within. I needed to open my heart because there was no doorknob on the outside which would allow someone access; everything I desire comes from within me. Upon this realization, my heart did begin to open and my tears would not stop. This release continued for twenty minutes or more and after this processing my whole body shook.

When you are looking at what your heart desires, know it could be standing outside your door but until you open the door to greater understanding and love, you will not see or receive it. The Life Tool: Violet Light Activation and Opening of the Heart, gently shows how to reach inside your heart to open the door. I suggest that after completing this process you energetically stand aside. What is coming in is huge, delightful and loving, so give it a wide berth and then enjoy it.

Life Tool: Opening of the Heart

Held within your heart are qualities to empower you. Here you will find the divine aspects of love, wisdom and power. Once these accolades are accessed the heart will open and be ready to receive the gifts which have been stored in your energy field for eons of time.

1.	Take a few deep cleansing breaths.
2.	Allow your body to relax and sink into a quiet space.
3.	Imagine yourself getting so small you could step into your physical heart.
4.	Move into one chamber within your heart and sense a light around you.
5.	The light transforms into a flame of three distinct colors: pink, yellow and blue.
6.	The pink represents the love within all life. With each breath allow the pink flame to expand and increase this love in your heart.

7.	The blue extension of the flame represents a higher essence of power.
	    a. This power holds no control; it stands upon a strength of its own and it is sharing it with you at this time.
	    b. Take time to feel this power and know it is real and easily accessed.

8.	The yellow flame is your inherent wisdom. This is knowledge beyond anything you have read or heard. It is the basis of your true inner understanding. Notice how it feels different than the other flames.
9.	Take a moment to receive and embody these qualities and notice how your awareness is enhanced.
10.	Step out of this flame while holding these qualities within your being.
11.	You are now standing at the door to your heart.
12.	Reach out and push the door open.
13.	On the outside is all that your heart desires.
14.	Imagine what it feels like to have these things in your life. This sensation empowers your dreams to manifest and become a reality.
15.	Complete your meditation with a sense of deep gratitude.

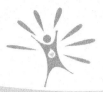

Manifestation Meditation

Focusing on the Reiki symbols while in meditation will increase their capacity each and every time you use them. The time spent visualizing each symbol will intensify their individual qualities which can be noticed the next time they are drawn. Your quiet attention to Reiki will send a message to your guides that you are serious about your practice and they will respond by giving you more assistance. Guides work with the higher self of the master and the master's clients. This can bring to the forefront information which could be used in the near future or for answers to a puzzling question. Once an idea is given form in the conscious mind through meditation, the subconscious mind will put the request into action. The symbols will help to locate and balance any imperfections held in the mind or body.

Each symbol will be imagined one by one, giving each symbol about ten minutes to stay in the stillness of the mind while recalling their visual image. After the time has elapsed allow the first symbol to float up, above your head, into a field of light. Do the same for the other traditional symbols. When all four symbols have been focused upon and illumined above your head, a desire may be empowered by these images.

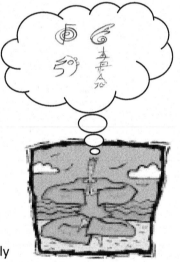

Be as specific as you can when forming your desire. It should appear in its completion with a sense of gratitude emanating from your heart. Keep this manifestation open ended so the Universe may fulfill the parts which will bring in the element of surprise and joy. The fun of receiving a gift is when you do not know exactly how it will appear and what it might hold for you.

 Remember: You will empower your desire by the feeling of manifesting it.

Once the picture of your desire is in your mind focus on how it feels to have this in your life. Imagine owning it, sharing it, touching it and being happy that you have it. That is where the power of manifestation lies. Feel as if it is already there, because it is; you have just not opened up to it yet. But you will after this meditation.

 Life Tool: Activating Symbols

The Reiki symbols can be intensified when they are visualized and anchored into your energy field. During this meditation, hold the master crystal from your crystal energy grid to empower it. The energy from the meditation will then be transferred into the stone, thus empowering the crystal energy grid the next time you charge it.

1.	Quiet the mind by taking three deep cleansing breaths.
a.	Listen to the rhythm of your breath.
b.	Call in and activate the Universal life force which surrounds every living thing. Drop into the feeling of this space.
2.	Draw the master symbol with your hand, imagining it as a laser beam of white or violet light.
a.	Close your eyes and visualize the symbol in your mind's eye.
b.	Stay in this quiet state until you feel the process is complete; this is usually about ten minutes.
c.	Then allow Dai-Ko-Mio to float above your head into a field of light.
3.	Repeat steps #1 to #2 with the following symbols:
a.	Power symbol, Cho-Ku-Rei.
b.	Mental and Emotional symbol, Sei-He-Ki.
c.	Distant symbol, Hon-Sha-Ze-Sho-Nen.
4.	The mind is now centered and positively charged.
5.	If time permits, empower a visualization with Manifesting Goals, it will
a.	Clearly manifest desires.

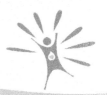

b.	Activate goals.
c.	Bring continued healing to others at a distance.

After meditating with the Reiki symbols, during your silent focus, the connection to your Reiki guides will be very strong and their knowledge will greatly empower any manifestation you request. So take a few more minutes and envision something you would like to manifest in your life or the life of another. See this picture fully complete and the laurels being received from its creation. There is no need to figure out how it can be accomplished; the Universe will fill in those gaps. Contact the feeling of how it is to have this accomplishment in your life for the emotion is what gives it power to manifest. This is a very important part.

When the meditation is complete, it is not necessary to make a similar request again in your next meditation. This will only negate the trust one has in knowing that the intent is already in motion. In a future meditation after focusing on the symbols as instructed previously, you may look in on the request; this is perfectly acceptable.

During this viewing you can check for the clarity of the vision and its proximity to the self. If it appears foggy, ask the guides to make it clearer. Sometimes the intent may seem far away and can be drawn closer while at other times the distance means it needs more time to process. While it is in the distant cosmos it will be magnetically drawing to itself people and situations which will empower it. Be at peace in your mind as you allow it to perform these feats. When an image is very close it can mean it will soon come into your life; just watch its movement without judgment. In the succeeding meditations, contact the feeling of having what you desire. It is the emotion which gives the intent momentum.

To complete the meditation you may embody the requested gift by anchoring it into the physical body at the "dan tien" also called the "tan tien," found just behind the navel.

The dan tien is spoken of in T'ai Chi and other eastern philosophies as a focus of power and the balancing center in the body. When the intent is directed to this spot in the body, the desire becomes solid. Physically draw your attention to this spot by gently tapping upon it.

There are three "L's" to mastery:

1.	**Learn** – read new material, practice the exercises and apply and use the many tools at your disposal.
2.	**Listen** – to your inner voice, let no one redirect your attention, this is your truth.
3.	**Let go** – release all the knowledge you have acquired and blaze your own path.

 Life Tool: Manifesting Goals

1.	If there is a crystal energy grid on the premises, meditate with the master crystal and then activate the grid with the stone at the end of the meditation.
2.	Clearly have a goal in mind or write it on paper.
	a. Visualize your personal desire or the intent for a client.
	b. For healing of another, imagine them in perfect health.
	c. For repair of an organ, see it functioning perfectly or transplant a new organ into its place.
	d. For emotional healing, imagine the individual enfolded in love and with an open heart receiving that love.
3.	Picture in your mind's eye the desire fully accomplished.
4.	Contact the feeling of obtaining this gift.
	a. Within the feeling is the power of manifestation.

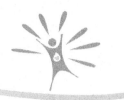

	b. Let go of the details required for its accomplishment; Spirit already has a plan.
	c. Spirit will fulfill your desires beyond your expectations.
5.	Hold the sensation of your desire in your mind and body and allow it to ascend into the light above your head, with the activated symbols.
6.	Do not ask for this wish again for it is accomplished on the first attempt.
7.	Visit the idea in meditation and feel how it has changed or become closer. Take time to notice what you perceive on an intuitive level.
8.	Trust your desire has been fulfilled and will materialize in divine time.
9.	Send the power from your head into the dan tien; the reservoir of power just below the navel.
10.	Tap on this area to activate and ground your desire.
11.	Take a long slow deep breath, slowly open your eyes and feel completely refreshed.

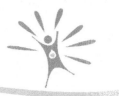

Chapter 6

Chakras

In order to be aware of what is happening in the world around you, you need to be cognizant of changes happening within your physical body first. When you are aware of accessing information through your body via your chakras, you will be able to respond quickly and accurately to situations happening daily. These centers help to interpret what you perceive as reality outside of your body, as you bring information into your body via these points. You are already receiving constant information from these power centers but may not be aware of how they communicate, thus missing their messages.

Various parts of your body process information differently. You are aware that your eyes and ears physically receive data, and the right and left sides of your brain access creative and analytical knowledge, but there are other parts of your body which process and receive information as well. In this chapter we will explore the myriad of ways these mysterious centers are attempting to get our attention.

Chakras and the DNA

Chakras are energy centers. They attach at the spine and extend out in front of the body in a cone shape; they allow us to interpret the apparent reality which appears before us. Not all information is accessed through sight and hearing. Emotions can be felt in the solar plexus by excitement causing the sensation of butterflies in the stomach, nausea occurring at the sight of gory images and actual pain when detrimental words are directed towards us. A lump in the throat will be felt when words are difficult to express, yet medically nothing can be detected as out of balance in the neck. All of these experiences are ways the chakras are directing information through the body.

In the past chakras have been described as wheels which spin in a clockwise direction, but this is not always be the case. As the earth raises her vibration, we ascend along with her. Our energy bodies and chakras therefore must change to accommodate the new vibrational frequencies. These changes are reflected in many aspects of the spiritual, mental and emotional bodies. Do not always expect these bodies to act as they have in the past. We are all individuals, and as we claim our differences, those qualities can be seen by activating new blueprints in the chakras. Change is evident, so when a chakra moves differently than in a spinning circle, ask if adjustments need to be made before assuming the chakra is out of balance.

Healing is associated with the medical profession and even their logo suggests that change can happen deep within the body. Its origin is equated with the ancient caduceus, the image is a double serpent entwined over the staff of the Greco-Roman god Hermes. The rod of Asclepius was the symbol of the Greek god of healing. Through the image of the intertwined snakes, this design reflects the DNA spiral. The wings over the snake suggest healing through divine intervention. Understanding how information is transferred and the depth of transformation which happens through the ancestral line in the DNA makes this symbol even more compelling.

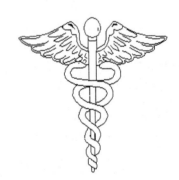

Medical caduceus reflecting
the DNA spiral

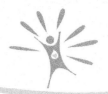

When a chakra does not follow the normal clockwise spin it may not be reflecting a need for change; it may be tuned into a new frequency, one that the person is aligning to. Some have observed the chakras as turning spheres or gears, rather than flat wheels. Each orb twirls in opposite directions and as they whirl they mirror a DNA spiral. This reflection of our DNA can be seen illustrated in the image which is an overlay on *The Vitruvian Man,* created by Leonardo da Vinci. By being aware of these new adjustments in the chakras, when you adjust and clear them, the transition will affect the DNA, making permanent changes all the way through the genetic line of the client. This especially happens when these shifts are anchored in the subconscious mind while you direct the client in a guided imagery meditation or hypnosis. Do not under estimate the power of your mind. When you visualize a change and empower it with your feelings, it happens, instantaneously.

You may begin a healing session may begin by checking the spin of the chakras of the client with the use of a pendulum or intuitive sight. Make the proper adjustments by directing energy into those energy centers and opening them to receive divine light. When checking the spin of a chakra, ask the higher self of the client if this center needs correction or if it is balanced in its diversity.

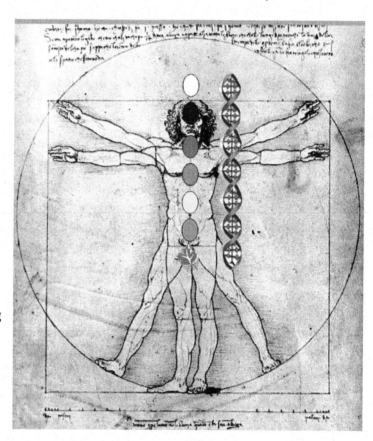

Chakras reflecting DNA spiral

Healing work on the planet has advanced to a point where it now has the ability to clear deep core issues, ones that have been handed down from generation to generation. These traumas are locked in the genetic coding of the body and when the client is supported with the love of Reiki, they will have the power to release them and it will make a lasting change for their entire family.

We are in constant change and growth, as are our chakras. Chakras continually cycle, and these patterns are explained by Cindi Dale in *New Chakra Healing*. Dale is a medical intuitive and has seen the chakras go through a different cycle every seven years, allowing an individual a chance to progress through each phase of their life. The change happens not only physically, but mentally and emotionally as well. When presented with these growth cycles, clients may release their judgments of themselves, seeing their challenges as part of their advancement in life rather than a hindrance. Look at the back of chapter four in Dale's book to see how these cycles apply to your age and chakra cycles. As we learn to understand ourselves and integrate our life processes, we can assist others to accept their seeming limitations in a new light.

Be aware of how you perceive the chakras in different clients for there is no one and only right way to sense these etheric bodies of light. They are as unique as the people you encounter. Tune into the individual process of the chakras for your client and make sure the chakras are aligned for that individual. Trust your instincts, honor what you see and do not second guess your intuition and abilities.

When a chakra is calling for attention you may help them balance this area of their body with one of the following meditations. The change will be lasting because the client will enter their subconscious mind through these deep relaxations. This is similar to the model used in hypnosis. The client is always in control and aware of what is being said by the hypno-therapist. The person who has been hypnotized will not do or say anything they would not normally say or do. Tell your client they may rest at ease because the same is true when we guide them in meditation.

When the mind is allowed to rest in this fashion, it contacts the subconscious, where long-lasting results occur. The conscious mind is a robot, run by the subconscious mind. Once the subconscious mind is entered, it can be redirected to serve the subject in a balanced and positive way.

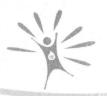

 Life Tool: The Red Base Chakra

Use this tool when finances are being a challenge and to receive manifestations of physical items such as a house, car, vacation, money, clothing and all things physical.

1.	Sit quietly in a chair, take three deep cleansing breaths and allow stillness to flow over your body.
2.	Imagine peace entering your body at your base chakra. It enters at the perineum, which is located between the genitals and the anus.
3.	Let the peace flow like a cool breeze and imagine this sensation entering your body.
4.	Allow the cool air to fill this entire space all the way up to the hip bones.
5.	Spend a little time relaxing into these sensations.
	a. If you are feeling nothing, make up a sensation.
	b. When you make believe, you are priming the pump of your imagination and creating a space for an actual felt activation.
6.	Concentrate on what you would like to physically manifest in your life.
7.	Think about how it would feel to acquire this.
8.	Visually see this gift you desire moving into this chakra center.
9.	Allow your body to house this desire.
10.	Receive, feel, sense and be grateful for the manifestation of your intention.
11.	See your plan already accomplished and offer gratitude for it. The key is to feel its energy blending with your energy.
12.	Revisit this new phenomenon once each day for the next three weeks.
	a. Watch its energy and see how it changes and adjusts. Give it time, for it takes 21 days to create or change a habit.
	b. Sense the integration of what you are manifesting.
13.	Take a deep breath, open your eyes and feel confident that you have already received your physical gift.

Life Tool: Orange Sacral Chakra

This center is where you will become aware of and activate your creativity. Focus on an area of your life that you feel could profit from a new idea. Then enter into the stillness of this meditation.

1.	Locate a quiet place where you will be undisturbed; turn off the phone.
2.	Allow your breath to slow down and deepen.
a.	Inhale through your nose.
b.	Exhale out through your mouth, making an audible sigh.
c.	Do this three times.
3.	Relax your forehead, your eyelids, your cheeks, your lips and your tongue.
4.	Allow this relaxation to penetrate across your face and into your head.
5.	Let it flow directly into your brain.
a.	From that point it streams down your entire body.
b.	Track it as it moves; notice the sensation it brings to various parts of your physical form.
6.	In your mind's eye pretend to step into the left side of your brain.
a.	This is the analytical side where you will allow your thoughts to just flow without focusing on any one idea.
b.	Attention here will allow the chatter to disperse as you give the mind time to let these ideas move through. Honor the way your left brain processes thoughts.
7.	Pretend to stand up and move to the creative right side of your brain.
8.	Take off your shoes and walk on the soft carpet.
a.	Sit on the velvet pillow on the floor.
b.	Feel the cool breeze coming in the window and the warmth of the sun or the coolness in the air. You design it.
c.	Notice how this side feels different from the left side.

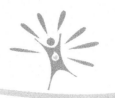

9.	Move to the center of your brain and remove any barriers you see here so you many integrate and feel the blending of the qualities of each side of your brain.
10.	You are now ready to access your creativity. Move your attention to your orange energy center just below your navel.
11.	Take a creative desire you have and plant it in the dirt.
12.	See warm yellow sunlight shining down on this subject matter from your chakra above.
13.	Watch it sprout and grow into a large plant.
14.	Sit beside this idea plant and receive the information it has stored inside.
	a. Watch for metaphors in this vision which will be clues to help construct this idea.
	b. The message may be revealed by the type of plant it becomes.
	c. The answer could come at a later time. Just know that the information has roots, it is growing and in time you will receive more about this message.
15.	Take a seed from this plant and place it in your throat chakra where it will grow and allow you to put this desire into action with your spoken word.
16.	When this process feels complete become aware of the sounds in the room, take a deep breath and open your eyes.

 Life Tool: The Yellow Solar Plexus Chakra

This center is the seat of your emotions. As you peer into this chakra do not place judgment on these sentiments by describing them as good or bad; accept each one for the value and balance they bring to you. In this tool, you will have an opportunity to uncover, greet, understand and make peace with emotions that have been locked away.

1.	Sit in a comfortable position.
a.	Loosen any tight clothing.
b.	Breathe slowly.
c.	Focus on the sound of your breath.
2.	Imagine your whole body moving with the rise and fall of your chest.
3.	Let this movement take you back to a time when you were being nurtured, lying in your mother's arms when she was rocking you. Even if you have no memory of this happening, allow it to occur in your mind's eye now and embrace your inner child.
4.	Let the sense of rocking move into your yellow energy center. The location is in your stomach, an inch and a half above your navel.
5.	Allow the rocking to change to waves on a gently flowing river.
6.	This river is the stream of your emotions and you are moving through it in a boat.
7.	There will be something appearing in the river which represents an emotion you are currently facing.
8.	If more than one emotion appears, acknowledge one and allow the other emotions to continue flowing down the river.
9.	Move your boat towards the emotion in whatever form it appears and confront it by looking straight into it.
10.	Know that you cannot be harmed by this emotion; it is only energy and you are empowered by facing it, rather than running from it.
11.	Ask it questions and receive the guidance it is holding for you.
12.	There is no need to rid an emotion from your body. Every sentiment, even the seemingly negative ones, has merit.
13.	This is your opportunity to discover the gift in all of your emotions. Bring them out of hiding and into the light and know they can no longer control you.
14.	Follow #9 to #13 with other emotions which surface from the waters.
15.	When you feel complete with the information received, allow your boat to once again travel along the river.

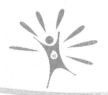

16.	Your boat glides to the shore and you step out and onto a beach.
17.	Feel your feet in the sandy soil. It is wet, cool and comforting.
18.	Sense your connection to the earth and anchor your new awareness into her. Feel the nurturing love of mother earth radiating into your body.
19.	When you feel complete with this process, take a deep breath and slowly open your eyes.

 Life Tool: The Green Heart Chakra

Sit quietly and allow your energy to drift into your center. Feel the movement in your chest as your breath carries you to this sacred place. Look into your heart and locate a place that feels comfortable. This is the place where you can begin to nurture yourself. One client observed mirrors when she entered her heart. This reflected the knowledge that her heart holds self-love. Every person in our lives in some way is reflecting back to us what we are projecting out.

1.	Light a candle, burn incense or bring in fresh cut flowers and enjoy their scent; this will awaken the right side of your brain.
2.	Sit on a pillow or chair and close your eyes.
3.	Begin to breathe slowly, noticing how the air enters your lungs as they gently rise and fall with each breath.
4.	Deepen your breath and allow your chest to expand as the air intake is increased, reflecting an opening of this center.
5.	On your exhalation, push all the old stale air out of your chest by letting your lungs drop and pulling your stomach in toward your spine.
6.	Repeat this deep breathing, bringing in and releasing as much air as possible. After the third breath relax and breathe normally.
7.	Remember someone, something or sometime where you felt love: the birth of a baby, a new puppy, falling in love or the awe of nature.

8.	Revisit how it felt in your body.
	a. Find the location in your body which holds the most sensation: is it inside, outside or in a chakra?
	b. How do you sense this feeling: do you see it physically, imagine it mentally or is it emotionally charged?
	c. It could merely be a sensation that is activated, but cannot be identified. This lets you become aware of how you intuit information.
9.	Sit in this energy and be aware of any changing sensations for a few minutes.
10.	Allow the feeling of love to move onto your skin and penetrate into your blood stream. Give it a color and perhaps a shape: a pink heart, a blue bubble, a golden stream.
11.	Love is being pumped in and out of your heart through the arteries. Notice if there is any resistance in a particular place in your body. Just observe it.
12.	Receive love as the blood pumps into your heart; extend this love out to yourself as the blood flows out of your heart.
13.	Feel this imagined sensation of love flowing through your entire body.
14.	Allow the image of love to pool in one chamber in your heart.
15.	Inside your heart, notice if you are alone.
	a. You may meet your inner child; acknowledge them.
	b. If heartache or sadness comes to mind, sit with it until it passes and allow the emotion to move or change.
16.	Whatever reaction arises from your heart, be present with the sentiment without analyzing it or even naming it.
	a. Do not judge it as good or bad; just honor it and stay with it.
	b. Do not leave it until you sense an integration of the uncovered concern.
17.	Notice if there is another aspect of yourself which appears that calls for your attention. If so, acknowledge it, release any judgment about it, love it and then blend and integrate with it.
18.	When you feel the process is complete, open your eyes and breathe in gratitude for the love which constantly flows through your entire body.

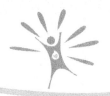

 Life Tool: The Blue Chakra

Within your throat is the power to manifest your heart's desires through your spoken words. Here you can see and release your unrealized fears that are holding you back from living a fulfilled life. Your dreams will only materialize when your thoughts are clear and the doorway to your manifestations is unobstructed. Being in touch with this energy center will support your wish.

1.	Sit quietly and close your eyes; see before you the beautiful aqua blue water of an island paradise.
2.	Walk or dive into the blue of this sea; immerse yourself safely within it.
3.	Let the blue flow into your throat and intensify.
4.	Place into the blue color, one of your heartfelt desires.
5.	Ask that one fear connected to this ambition arise.
	a. Allow it to surface from the sea.
	b. It may manifest as a feeling, a color, an image or a story.
6.	Become conscious of any sensations in your throat, in your body or outside your body as you proceed in this exercise.
7.	Observe if there is any information here you need to acquire about this fear. Then let it go by placing it in a bubble and see it floating off into the sky.
8.	Invite another fear to present itself before you in the water.
	a. Follow steps #6 to #9.
	b. Continue until your fears about this desire no longer surface.
9.	Once all fears are released, revisit your heart's desire. Does it look different?
10.	See your desire already accomplished and feel gratitude for it.
11.	Once again, notice the subtle sensations in your throat.
12.	Each time you use this exercise it can bring in different feelings. Do not judge their effectiveness. Allow each meditation to be its own experience.
13.	When you feel the process is complete, focus on your breath, allow it to deepen, then slowly and gently open your eyes as you feel a sense of accomplishment.

Life Tool: Indigo Chakra

Focusing within this center will open intuitive ideas and help clear the thoughts when you are unfocused and scattered. Become familiar with the feelings in this center while relaxed, so that when you need to access ideas, the process will be effortless.

1.	Begin by having no agenda or expectations for the outcome of this exercise. Request for clarification on an idea you have.
2.	Close your eyes place your finger on your forehead and rub in a circular motion.
3.	Remove your finger and continue to imagine the sensation.
4.	Let the circular motion move deeper into your forehead at the frontal lobes of your brain.
5.	Imagine scattered thoughts stirring around in your mind.
6.	Stop the swirling and look at the first thought that comes to your awareness. Is this your thought or does it belong to someone else?
7.	Let go of the imposed thoughts from others and meet with only your thoughts; do not force anything to happen.
8.	Be present with any sensations as they enter your consciousness.
9.	Information may be in the form of thoughts, feelings, visions or unexplained but obvious impressions.
10.	Stay with your feelings. When thoughts arise, stop the process of looking and just feel what they contain. This will move you out of your analytical mind and open you to receive the gift of your intuition.
11.	Maintain your energy in the deep blue purple color of your forehead.
12.	Notice what happens and if no further information is attained, know that a new insight will be presented in the next three days, so be consciously aware and watch for it in words or metaphors.
13.	The time just spent in this center has activated and increased your psychic abilities. As you come back into conscious awareness, affirm your new-found skills. Take a deep breath and open your eyes.

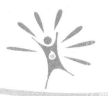

 Life Tool: White Chakra

At the very top of your head is your connection to the divine aspects of yourself and the divine which is present around all living things. There are no questions to be asked here. It is only a place for surrender. Trust is the word to focus upon; time does not exist here, as this Life Tool will move you outside of the time continuum.

1.	Align your body and mind into a comfortable place.
2.	Let your breath take you to a state of complete surrender.
	a. Yield to any ache or pain in the body.
	b. Give in to your thoughts. Let them flow. There is no agenda.
3.	Imagine a soft white light around your entire body.
4.	Ask for your divine essence to float up and into the light.
5.	Within this light, remember the sensation of love.
	a. It cannot be intellectualized, only felt.
	b. It will feel different each time you actualize it.
6.	Lift this love beyond human attributes and trust that you can fly into it.
7.	Feel yourself rising into the sky, past the earth's atmosphere and into the stars. Open to the awe of infinity; imagine nebulas and the beauty of the universe.
8.	Let this beauty support your spirit and dreams. There is no image here, only the feeling of movement and love.
9.	Sense that you are not alone. Ask for an image of love and support, which is always enfolding you in some way, to show its presence. Stay with it.
10.	Float in this timeless space until you are once again conscious of the earth.
11.	At the edge of the earth's atmosphere is a membrane, comprised of a protective love for the earth and her inhabitants. Touch it.
12.	Notice how palpable it feels; allow yourself to become fully aware of this area.
13.	When you are done exploring float back into your body and take a deep breath and sigh.
14.	Feel your feet firmly on the ground as you anchor the divine light of the cosmos into the earth and into every aspect of your life.

Each energy center is fed from the one below and guided from the one above; this is a natural progression. Through this energy highway flows an energetic electrical juice. It can also be seen as flames igniting and activating the Kundalini energy. The Sanskrit definition for Kundalini is "coiled" and this energy is seen as a sleeping serpent in the base chakra. Its awakening can be accomplished with the breath, with yoga movements or by the development of consciousness. The path of Reiki is a road to consciousness; therefore, when you follow the energy progression through the levels of Reiki, a sense of this awakening can be partially or even fully experienced. By focusing on how each chakra supports the other you can begin to activate this flow. When the analytical brain understands how the flow of Kundalini is accomplished it becomes appeased which then allows the sensations of the body to be fully opened.

How Adjacent Chakras Support Each Other

1.	The lowest red chakra brings in the nurturing energy of mother earth while it anchors the creative process of the orange center above.
2.	The orange center is fed by the emotions streaming from the yellow center, adding to its innovative nature. The red chakra below moves the creative energy into the earth for manifestation.
3.	The yellow emotional center is nourished by the imaginative orange center as the love in the heart balances and leads desires with passion.
4.	The green energy center of the heart has a foothold in the yellow emotional center to support and direct it so that harmony is embodied. The blue chakra above gives the power needed for materialization of any heart desired activities into motion via the voice.
5.	The blue energy center of power will not get far if not fueled by compassion in the heart chakra below. It is the discernment of the indigo center above the blue chakra that forms a beacon of light to advise the voice of the blue center.
6.	It is through the efficiency and power in the blue energy center that the indigo center is endowed with enough skill to accept the advice being sensed

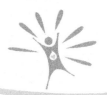

	as trust flows from the crown to feed these divine thoughts and allow them to manifest.
7.	The top white chakra, when focused upon, will inspire thoughts to come through to the highest degree. The white center connects to the highest essence of the divine self and holds the qualities of all the energy centers of the body. It has the ability to blend, discern, encourage and stabilize actions.

 Life Tool: Awakening the Kundalini

This Life Tool will gently open Kundalini energy. The Kundalini energy is dormant in the base of the spine until activated through the practice of yoga or conscious intent in meditation. When the shoots up through the body from the base chakra, all of the chakras will open and clear. This can be a gentle process when the individual holds the clear intent for it to be so. Each chakra is ignited and encouraged to light the chakra above until they are all blend into an iridescent light at the crown of the head.

1.	Locate a quiet place; sit and breathe slowly as you let your muscles relax.
2.	Imagine your base chakra, located at the tailbone, as a red flame. Create a sensation in this center which reminds you of a warm, glowing fireplace.
3.	Let the tip grow and ignite the orange flame above, just below the navel.
4.	The red flame enfolds the orange and continues to grow. Allow the warmth of the red flame to embrace creative ideas, which are ready to blaze into your awareness. Feel it.
5.	The orange/red flame expands and lights the yellow flame at your stomach. Disturbing emotions begin to melt into the warmth as fear and stress begin to dissolve away.
6.	The combined flame grows taller and activates the green flame in your heart. Allow your breath to deepen and expand your lungs to make room for this opening to this center of love.
7.	As your heart's love grows, it touches the blue flame in your throat. Love enfolds and softens the power being unleashed in this center. Notice if it holds a particular sensation for you at this time.

8.	The blue flame extends up to light the indigo flame at the forehead. The power from the blue light activates not only clarity within the indigo flame but the assurance of knowing your psychic powers as well.
9.	The indigo flame is clear and bright and it extends through the top of the head. It turns into an iridescent white flame, which is a combination of all the colors of your chakras.
10.	The colors blend and enfold all positive qualities from the earth, the sky and your divine being.
11.	At the top of your head, all the flames blend into one powerful, colorful flame. Feel the power of the combined energy of your chakras.
12.	Imagine before you a doorway. Center yourself before you walk through it, for this is where you will claim your power and embody your divine essence.
13.	Once inside let go of your thoughts and just be with the feeling of resonating at this high frequency.
14.	Take time to become acquainted with a new way of seeing yourself: confident, strong and self-assured.
15.	From here you can view your life options in a new way. Relax in this space until you once again become aware of your breath.
16.	Walk back out of the doorway.
17.	Imagine moving into your body, down from your head to your forehead.
18.	The color is a beautifully clear indigo.
19.	Descend through the blue power in your throat.
20.	Continue moving as you drop into the soft green of your heart.
21.	Drop through the yellow in your emotional chakra at your stomach.
22.	Sense your increased creativity in the orange chakra.
23.	You are back in your room as you imagine the red around your tailbone.
24.	On the count of three, you will open your eyes and feel totally refreshed.
25.	Now you have started to shift your energy.
26.	You know what it feels like to vibrate at the frequency that supports self love and gives you self-confidence.

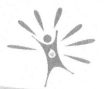

Chakra Vortices

Each chakra often spins in a clockwise direction and within these whirls are numerous vortices. The number increases with each ascending chakra until it reaches the crown, which seats 972 vortices. The crown chakra has often been referred to as the thousand-petaled lotus. This alludes to the individual whirlpools within the crown. For simplicity, the number is rounded up to 1000.

Through the chakras, energy moves into the blood, it can travel very quickly to any place that needs balance. This is how Reiki and other energy modalities can move to the area of the body which is in need. Because part of the energy transfer is directed through the endocrine glands, traditional Reiki has the practitioner hold hand positions only over these glands. Each chakra corresponds to a specific endocrine gland, noted as follows:

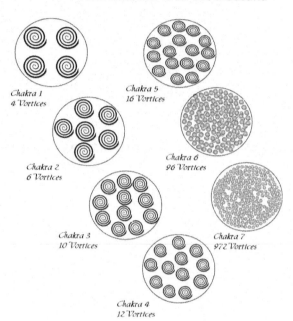

Chakra 1
4 Vortices

Chakra 2
6 Vortices

Chakra 3
10 Vortices

Chakra 4
12 Vortices

Chakra 5
16 Vortices

Chakra 6
96 Vortices

Chakra 7
972 Vortices

Chakra	Endocrine Gland	# of Spinning Vortices
#7 Crown:	Pineal	972
#6 Third Eye:	Pituitary	96
#5 Throat:	Thyroid	16
#4 Heart	Thymus	12
#3 Solar Plexus	Pancreas	10
#2 Sacral	Gonads	6
#1 Base	Adrenals	4

Number of vortices contained within each chakra

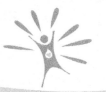

Chapter 7

Advanced Techniques

Your intuitive abilities will increase as you advance with each level of Reiki. Because nontraditional Reiki encourages one to use Reiki on a daily basis in every walk of life rather than keeping this energy for treatment sessions only, the following practices will come in handy. You may find the skill of reading auras will be your quick way to interpret the energies of others. This will be advantageous as it could show you how to proceed in a business meeting, while conducting sales, and in almost any relationship situation. These skills do not require quiet concentration for they can be practiced in a public setting without anyone around you knowing what you're doing.

The Life Tool: Energetic Release will allow any disturbance in the body to be revealed and released as it is given a form. This moves emotions and pain from the esoteric realm where they are difficult to grasp to a place where they can be seen and easily worked with. Because the client will be supported by the master's high intuitive abilities the client will also be able to view the form that their old issues hold. The client can then see their discomfort change, transform and leave. This becomes a very powerful tool.

Sensing Auras

Developing the skill to see auras can be fun, but do not put too much stock in what you see. The human aura adapts quickly to what is sensed in and around it, therefore it is not stable. It changes according to personal thoughts, influences of others and activities in the environment. Even the breathing pattern of the person you are watching will influence its size and shape. The colors of an aura will change as fast as a thought, so use this practice to develop your inner sight and have fun doing it but know that what you see will not always give clear insight to the subject. You intuition will be a better mark.

The best way to see the energy radiating from the body is to have the subject sit or stand in front of a lightly colored wall in a naturally lit room. Standing outside in direct sun light will wash out the colors of the aura, while florescent light is not a good choice because a florescent bulb is constantly pulsing which can be stressful to the eyes. Though candle light works well, watch that the candle does not cast shadows on the background behind the subject.

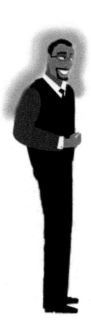

Stand back about six to ten feet from your subject and focus on the wall behind their body. Then change your focus to view the air which occupies the space between the subject and the wall. The area which you will first notice will be about an inch or two off their head or shoulders. You may softly focus your eyes so images appear fuzzy to aid in the viewing of the aura. If you wear glasses, remove them as this will have the same effect. Look at your subject with a soft stare. The challenge lies in holding the soft focus and not allowing the eyes to revert back to normal viewing. Pay attention to your thoughts as the aura will disappear as soon as you begin to doubt what you are seeing.

Normal Aura

The aura will at first appear very subtle and you may question if you are actually seeing it or if this is only a figment of your imagination. The aura can also appear to drift in and out. This is your conscious mind trying to make sense

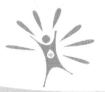

out of what you are seeing. As you silence your left brain and allow your right brain to take over, the process will become easier. Over the years we have had very few opportunities to develop our inner sight; in fact most of the time it has been denied by society. The mind is recalling that pattern, so give it time to adjust to a new way of thinking and soon this natural ability will be recalled again and empowered.

Once you have established that you are seeing the etheric body, ask the subject to breathe slowly and deeply. Watch the fuzzy grey outline or white envelope expand and contract as they change the rhythm of their breath. This envelope can be easily seen off the head and shoulders and with practice it can be viewed around the entire body. Suggest that your subject rock from side to side. It will then be easy to see their aura move with them as it slightly lags behind.

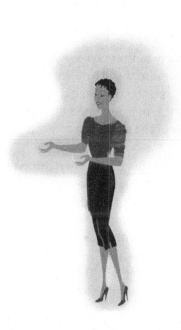

When you become accustomed to viewing the aura with a light background, have the subject move in front of a dark wall. Soften your stare once again and focus your gaze an inch or two off their body, directing your view to the wall. Look at the air between the subject and the background behind them. The haze will once again appear.

While viewing the subject's aura is being viewed, have them turn the palms of their hands up and place your hands over theirs; do not touch them, only channel Reiki or energy into them. The aura will begin to change and grow. Another technique is to step back and ask them to think of someone they love. Watch the change. Then ask them to think of other emotions, such as anger, peace, sadness, joy, guilt, and contentment. Notice the change as they go from positive to negative thoughts.

Remembering positive emotions
  increases the size of the aura.

If the subject breathes fast, it will increase the size of the aura, while slowing their breath will actually make it shrink. Watch people regularly with this simple technique to increase your ability and to fill the time while you are at the airport, standing in line at the store, sitting in an office or waiting for the lights to dim at the movie theater. The amount of time given to practicing will greatly increase your skill in seeing auras.

To view your own aura, stand in front of a mirror while using the techniques described above. Use different colored backgrounds and try rocking from side to side and watch your aura follow you. Remember different emotions or people in your life. Can you see the change?

Once the energy can be easily viewed, begin to look for the color of the aura. At first you may not see a color but observe your thoughts and see if you have a sense of a color or an idea of a color that enters your mind. After you acknowledge this thought, the color will often appear.

Example: As I watch performers on stage I find that many of them have a beautiful purple glow. This is the color of the crown chakra; it is where the artists' inspiration originates and the area where most entertainers are connected to while they channel the light of their higher essence during their performance. In a darkened theater, it is very easy to see their auras appear as well as the auras of those in the audience.

The aura has a vibration which is almost easier to detect in the dark. When the eyes are allowed to ease into the darkness by slowly turning down the lights the aura magically pops out. Begin this exercise in a room equipped with a dimmer for the lighting. Stand as far apart from your subject as the room permits and look at their aura. Once the aura is detected, slowly dim the lights and notice how bright the aura becomes. Your eyes will adjust to the softness of the light and even with the lights low, the aura will still be apparent; in fact it intensifies once the lights are completely turned off. This can be a fun activity to try with friends and family because anyone can acquire the skill to view auras.

Not only can auras be seen but the energy in the air around us can also be observed rather easily. Barbara Brennan, in her book *Hands of Light,* refers to energy squiggles that can be seen by looking into the air[4]. They are easily visible outside on a sunny day or inside while focusing on the light above a lamp. This is good training for releasing the

---

[4] Barbara Brennan. *Hands of Light,* 39

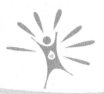

doubt held in the analytical mind of the left brain. Focus your eyes into the light about ten feet from your body and up at a 45 degree angle. You are really looking at nothing as you gaze into the air and observe what appears. The energy squiggles will dart from place to place and emerge in a matter of a minute or two. By developing this technique, you will find the practice of seeing auras easier as the veil between dimensions dissolve.

Aura Colors

The following are possible meanings for the colors seen and sensed in the aura. These are only guidelines; the information perceived by the viewer should always be honored first, for that is the activation of their inner sight and intuition, which they should heed. The subject will be subconsciously directing information through the colors of their auras, guiding the viewer to these deeper insights. Listen first to your feelings rather than always giving credence to the intellect. The following list is one person's observations at a given time with their subjects. You may pick up different information when you are viewing an aura. Honor your intuitive thoughts and the information you are being given by the subject and what their colors mean for them that day.

Aura Colors and their Meanings

Purple	Spiritual, connecting with God, mystic seeing and cosmic connections.
Indigo	Wisdom, intuition, spirituality and spiritual personality, artistic tendency, self empowerment and being in harmony with nature.
Blue	Psychic power, intelligence and logical thinking.
Lt. Blue	Strong intuitive capabilities.
Dk. Blue	Strong, analytical and suspicious personality.
Green	Balance, healing, finding peace and harmony.
Lt. Green	Ability to be compatible with lots of things.
Dk. Green	Jealousy, as though green with envy.
Yellow	Love, kindness, compassion and openness, and the breath of life.

Dk. Yellow	Greediness, suspicion.
Orange	Energy and health, physical vitality, dynamic personality and an overabundance of self-righteousness.
Dk. Orange	Lower intelligence.
Red	Closer to the physical body, vitality, sexual energy and ambition.
Dark Red Scarlet	Aggressions, anger, focus located in the sexual organs, materialism and lower insights.
Pink	Unselfish love.
Brown	Selfish, greedy, looking for profits out of a situation and manipulative.
Gold	Higher consciousness, good personality and harmony.
Silver	Energy and constant changes.

Developing your skill to look at auras is just another way to heighten your intuition. Each exercise practiced will let you know which way you can best sense information in an aura. The master's abilities shine when they know various ways to peer into the unseen bodies of a client. The individuality of each client and the master makes a variety of techniques a necessity. Always honor your inner gifts as you apply the processes given. This is just one more tool you can place in your energetic tool box.

Spirits in the Aura

When darkened forms appear in the aura they may not be negative intruders but could be ones with information for their host. There is undoubtedly a reason for their presence and you have the ability to decipher this code.

 Remember: Spirits are just like people. They do not show up for a visit unless they have a reason to do so.

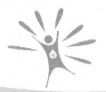

The spirit may have attached because it wanted to help someone understand their current situation, so it is not necessarily a bad thing. Addressing the form with compassion, love and curiosity will dispel any anger or assumed attack. If you feel the need, before you encounter this spirit, invite a higher level being or angel to stand by your side.

Example: I was called upon to investigate a spirit in a home in the Colorado mountains. Before I arrived I spoke with the owner and she told me about the numerous encounters she had had with this spirit. When she was not home it would mimic her voice and footsteps and call to the cleaning lady who never saw the source of the false voice. The spirit would also make its presence known by screaming and crying. This would of course upset the entire household. The owner could tell by its voice it was a small girl.

As I hung up the phone my first thought was, What am I doing going up to clear such an aggressive spirit? I am not qualified to do this. Then I allowed my mind to still and I dropped into my heart. I tuned to this small spirit and I could feel *her* fear. I spent the next few minutes assuring her I was coming to help her and she did not need to be afraid any more. I was going to help her find her mommy.

I treated this spirit just as I would if I found a little girl alone, crying and afraid. This dispelled not only my fear but hers as well. I approached the home with love in my heart and though it took almost two hours to completely clear this very large home it was not difficult or scary. The spirit needed time to trust me and process everything which was transpiring. She had been alone for years and it took time for her to adjust to someone actually speaking to her rather than running from her.

You can assist a spirit in someone's aura in a similar manner. They are not to be feared, they are just lonely, afraid and want to be understood. If they do things which scare their host it is because they are trying to get their attention.

What happens around us is our own creation. We have invited these energies into our space for a reason. It could be so they can help us or because they know we can help them, in any case we have opened the door to their realm. The spirit has some kind of knowledge so all we need to do is to ask for them to show us the information. The people who have hosted the seemingly uninvited guest could be angry about their continued presence and this agitation needs to be released. Calling in light beings and guides while attempting to receive information from a spirit will ease any resentment or fear the client may have, and soften them so they can understand the reason the spirit appeared in their energy field. As for this little girl, all she wanted was to go home. She was lonely and frightened and was asking the people in the house for help.

Talk to the spirit as you would any stranger who has entered a room. Find out why it has shown up and if it has a message for your client. When the spirit is resistant to sharing information, make it simple for it to respond. Tell it to bounce up and down for a yes response and back and forth for a no. Then proceed with questions which can be answered in this way. If it seems appropriate ask your client to view this questioning as well and see what they pick up. The spirit has called to them so they really are acquainted with its energy and can sometimes access information as well. The Life Tool: Transition to the Light in chapter 4 or the Life Tool: Releasing Spirit Attachments in chapter 3 of *Inner Gifts Uncovered* will give ideas as how to guide these beings out of this realm and onto their next path.

Energetic Release

Healing in this process comes from empowering the client to see how a physical or emotional issue has become a framework within their body or energy bodies. Negative energy can take on many different shapes, either around the organs, in the body or out in the aura. These models can block the incoming life force and create emotional and physical imbalances. During the energetic release, the client will be enveloped within the master's energy, which will allow the client to access their own image as to how their issue has taken form in and around their body. When a clairvoyant sees and informs a client of negative energy around their body, the truth of its presence can be rejected because it is not information discovered and seen by the client. Not so when such negative energy is envisioned and sensed by the client themselves. Therein lies the value of this process.

Emotions are so esoteric that they can easily be stuffed away and ignored. Giving the emotion a visual figure, makes it real, thus making it easier to release. I have had clients who have seen their heart issue as a heavy iron lung over their chest, back pain in the

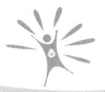

form of a snake entwined around their spine and the inability to speak their mind as a hand gripping their throat. When they redesigned the visual image it balanced and eased their mind and body.

Example: The client with the iron lung discovered they created it to protect and hide their heart from pain. By the client's design, it was changed into a beautiful gossamer veil which shadows and protects the client while still allowing the radiance of divine light to enter.

As for the snake that encompassed the spine, the client asked for it to change into a vine of roses. At first it had thorns which could still create pain, but when she asked for them to be removed, they quickly transformed. The client is empowered when they can see the changes happen by merely making a request.

In the last example, the grip of the hand was released and the client was able to speak her truth without fear of harming others. She replaced it with a lapis necklace which has the power to heal and support one in speaking their truth.

Help the client open their senses by asking questions that will prime the pump of their intuitive awareness. The answers are deeply locked within their psyche; as master, you will hold a sacred space for the client to see how they can heal themselves. This allows them to continue on this path of self-empowerment later on their own.

 Remember: Often the easiest image to sense will be color.

The process begins by assisting the client to see what form their physical or emotional issue has taken in their body. You will ask these simple questions, "If the issue had a color, what color it would be. What is the shape, texture, weight, smell and emotion they perceive?" The patron may not have an answer for each question, but as each inquiry is made, the intuition of the client increases. If no answer comes to mind have the client make up an answer. This will stimulate their visual process.

 Remember: Science has proven that the mind does not know the difference between imagination and reality: the brain waves are identical for both.

Let them know that even pretending to see an image will be beneficial in removing the stress associated with their dilemma. There are no wrong answers and each session will have a different twist than the one before. There was a client whose issue moved its location throughout their body periodically. It was running and trying to hide. We followed it and continued to ask questions. The profile changed many times before its true essence was revealed and then released, but the truth was eventually uncovered. Do not rush your client into clearing these issues. Allow them the time they need. With the divine light of Reiki everything is being cleared with love at its own pace, so hold a sacred space for your client and know all is happening in divine order.

Call for assistance from angels and guides when you become confused and unclear about the next step to take. This higher source will give information so that the process will evolve to the next level as the clearing occurs. Always ask for guidance from beings whose power and vibration are greater than what you hold at this time. When I get stuck, my guides have never failed me. My clients always leave the session with new perceptions and understandings. I have yet to see it fail.

Example: When I feel stuck and do not know the next step to take with my client I take a moment and still my thoughts and energy field. This occurs in a split second. I let the energy of love flow into my body, I ask for assistance from the divine light beings that are present for this session and I sense my connection to my divine intelligence. Clear direction then arrives in a matter of seconds.

The reason the client can visually see within their body with inner eyes is that they are under the umbrella of the master's energy. Under that radiance, they will see and sense more than they usually see on their own. The master brings in a very high frequency for guidance and divine love, which allows a new perception of the reoccurring issue to surface. The client will then have access to perceive this information. Allow them their own experience in this process; guide them but do not interfere with or negate their visions.

The client uncovers new perspectives while the master gently directs them while channeling the love of Reiki. In this area, compassion and knowledge exist. It is within the power of the master to hold the clear intent for the client to have total and precise understandings of the situation being addressed. This process empowers the client, allowing them to know that they have created what stands in their way and therefore

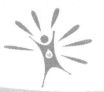

they have the ability to clear this obstacle and move forward. A true master will empower their client so the client will continue to do their own self-healing, without continually relying on the master for assistance.

Talking to the Form

Once the appearance of the issue has been discovered, the process begins. A dialogue is started between the client and the structure. The reason an ailment stays in the body is that there is a directive to be heard. Pain is one way the body gets attention. It creates discomfort so that the person will stop, listen and often receive new ways to look at old issues. The body is only a message center and many of these messages have been recorded in books which list physical ailments and the most common emotions tied to them. As mentioned before, Louise Hays, author of *Heal Your Body*, and Karol Truman, author of *Feelings Buried Alive Never Die*, both have published extensive information on this subject.

Guiding the client through the "energetic release" helps them begin to venture into the path of self-discovery. As the client uncovers their stories through the scenario they have created within themselves, they are empowered with the guidance of the Reiki master, to reveal their personal messages and begin their healing process.

Instruct the client to begin a conversation with the system perceived. Ask the form, "Why are you here? How have you helped me? Is there a message I need to hear?" Sometimes the client is afraid to let go of the figure because they think that in some way it is protecting them. In the case of the woman with the imagined iron lung, she claimed she could not remove the iron lung because it was necessary to shield her heart. She said, "If I take this off I will get hurt." I then informed her that she could change the design into another model which would not inflict pain, either emotionally or physically. This gave her permission to continue the release.

When the client is dialoguing with the perceived shape and there appears to be no response, tell them to pretend there is. "Fake it till you make it" gets the process moving. Make up a conversation until something happens which was not imagined by the one holding the conversation. By using the imagination, the client accesses real intuitive Eventually the client will perceive something and the actual reason for the discomfort in their body will be disclosed. Once discovered, the image no longer has reason to stay. It will diffuse often without direction, and a new figure, which serves the client's higher good, can be created to replace it.

Completely Removing the Image

Just finding and conversing with the form in the body it can begin to dissolve it, often without any direct assistance from the master. The dialogue is between the client and the image they have created in their own body which houses their physical or emotional pain. Once the client gleans information from this form, they will often open to see a new perception. This awareness moves them to feel compassion and love for what they have created, which allows the pattern to be easily released. When the client can see for themselves that the image is leaving, it becomes real to them. They are then empowered because they know they made it happen and they saw it transform. This becomes their truth and not something they have been told.

If the form perceived does not completely dissipate, continue to direct the patron to ask for information from the image until it totally dissolves. As long as there is the slightest wisp of the structure, there is knowledge to be received. Keep asking questions and stay on track until the client releases the image completely. When the silhouette is resistant to talking, imagine it to be an old friend, which it is. If the problem is chronic, then the client has housed it for many years and it has become an integral part of their makeup. Tell your client to pretend to begin a simple conversation: "Hello, my name is Tom, are you comfortable sitting in my stomach? I have abdominal pain; do you know what is causing this? Do you know how I can feel better? What do you need from me? I am listening, give me a clue; let's get started."

With each question, direct the client to imagine an answer; this will be done silently by the client or audibly if they choose. They can also ask it to respond by giving yes and no replies by moving up and down or back and forth. Allow the client to connect with this form on their own. After a few moments ask the client to share what is happening; this will keep them on track. Checking in with them periodically will keep the client present with the release so they will not drift off and lose track of what they are doing. What they share will assist you as the master to stay in the same direction they are going. Remember, this is their process; let them lead; the master merely holds the space and

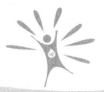

interjects guidance when needed.

The process clears the issue fully because when you are channeling Reiki to the client, they enter a subconscious state, similar to hypnosis. In this deeply relaxed state the subconscious mind is reprogrammed and the new perceptions will anchor into the conscious mind, creating a lasting change.

Any time something is removed that once held space in and around the body, if no direction is given, anything, positive or negative, can take its place. Therefore, the client needs to imagine a new model to take the place of the old encumbered one. The new image becomes real by the client's giving it form, color, shape, texture, scent and emotion. Once all these elements are in place, the metamorphosis will occur. By this time in the session the client has become so visual that when they are directed to place a new image in their body they will clearly describe it. If they do not, then you may ask them to give it color, form and texture. It is very important to remember to place a new form in the space of the old one or the effects of the process could diminish and the old issue might resurface.

There have been occasions when the body required time to clear before the new image could be installed. Perhaps this will be two or three days. In that case, have the client set up the new form near the area where the old image was. Once the area is clear, the prescribed object will integrate.

If the old issue resurfaces, the client can remember their process and affirm that the old figure has been replaced by a new object which will assist rather than perturb. Contacting all of the five senses of the new design will make its presence feel real. This will be done by giving the image a color, size, shape, texture, emotion and fragrance.

The higher self of the client will guide the master all along the way. If longer clearings are required, your intuition will make it known. You may use your pendulum to determine the length of time required for the clearing. You can ask, "How long will it take to integrate this process: minutes, hours, days or weeks?" You will find that most of the time the process will complete during the session.

Life Tool: Energetic Release

The important aspects while guiding the client through the process are underlined for quick reference. This will help so that the master can follow their personal guidance with little need to follow a prescribed script.

1.	Have the client identify the issue they would like to clear.
2.	Tell them you will help them give this issue form and when questions are presented to them, know that there are no wrong answers.
3.	Have the client lie on the massage table and place your hands on their body while you channel the divine light of Reiki.
4.	Draw the power symbol followed by the other traditional symbols.
5.	Accept your ability to hold a sacred space and intuit the guidance of their higher self.
6.	Ask the client, if this problem had a color, what <u>color</u> it would be.
	a. What <u>shape</u> does it hold?
	b. How heavy is it; what is its <u>weight</u>?
	c. What is the <u>texture</u>: smooth, rough, sticky?
	d. Is there a <u>sound</u> associated with it?
	e. Is there an <u>emotion</u> felt when connecting to it? How does it make you feel?
7.	<u>Where does it reside</u> near the body?
	a. Is it deep within?
	b. On the surface?
	c. Above the body?
	d. It may be in more than one place.
8.	Ask the client these pertinent questions:
	a. <u>Are you ready to release this form</u>? If the response is no, tell the client they can replace this form with another image which will not hurt or disturb them.
	b. <u>Are you open to receive information it may hold for you</u>?

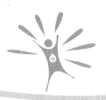

c.	Are you prepared to act on the information given?
9.	When you have received a positive response to these questions, permission is granted and the process is underway.
10.	Center your energy; ask for guidance from beings of equal or greater power than your own as well as the divine self of your client. Imagine connecting heart to heart with your client.
11.	Draw Cho-Ku-Rei over the area described.
12.	Send energy into the body until you feel it is time to ask the client to talk to the form. This will only be a few minutes.
13.	Have the client begin a conversation with the image. Start with small talk and then advance to the following questions:
a.	What is the reason for your visit? Can I help you?
b.	Have you been helping me? If so, how?
c.	Do you have a message to share?
14.	Let their conversation continue and as the client honors and blesses this form, it will usually begin to change and lighten.
15.	Once the answers are received, continue with these directives to the client:
a.	Give the form love, thanks and gratitude.
b.	Honor its existence and tell it you no longer need its presence.
c.	Tell it you are ready to release it now.
16.	As the client honors and blesses this image, it will begin to morph.
17.	Help the client stay with the process by asking what they see and sense is happening.
18.	If the shape does not completely clear, direct the client to continue a dialogue with the perceived form, searching to uncover helpful information.
19.	Once the figure is cleared you may complete the process.
20.	A void is created by removing the object, this area requires a new constructive item to be put in its place.
21.	It will be seen as real when the five senses are addressed. Ask the client:

a.	What would you like to put here in its place?
b.	What color is it?
c.	Describe the size, shape, texture, fragrance and emotion.
22.	Inform the client the next time they feel the pain or contact the emotion formally held in this image, recall the new model and all of its attributes.
23.	Finalize the session with a Reiki treatment.

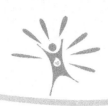

Life Tool: Energetic Release

Identify the problem.	Bring in Reiki, divine assistance and the Reiki symbols.	Find where the image resides.	Hold a sacred space while channeling in Reiki.
Ask questions about the form perceived.	What is the color?	Weight, shape, texture?	What is the emotion, sound or smell?
Where is it in the body?	Deep within?	On the surface?	Outside the body?
Ask the client:	Are you ready to release it?	Willing to receive information from it?	Prepared to act on the information given?
Ask the image:	What is the reason for your visit? Can I help you?	Are you here to help me? If so, how?	Do you have a message to share?
After information is received:	Give thanks to the image.	Tell the image thank you but its services are no longer required.	It will now be replaced by a constructive image.
Fill the void with a new form.	What color is it?	What is the size, shape and texture?	Give it an emotion and a fragrance.
Remind the client they now have a powerful image to draw from.	Complete the session with a full Reiki treatment.		

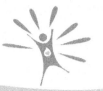

Chapter 8

Animals and Reiki

The basic Reiki technique used in healing is wonderful on its own but there is so much more that can be done with the channeled light of Reiki. In this chapter we are going to step out of the general understanding of Reiki and explore how to apply the transcendent love of Reiki to animals.

Pets greatly benefit from the energy of Reiki because they do not have the limits of our complex emotional bodies. True, they hold memories and if they were once abused they will carry that pain during their life but they are not bound by lifetimes of trauma. It is reassuring to apply the healing to them, as they are quite responsive, which always encourages the practitioner to continue in their practice. The presence you hold in your home radiates through the atmosphere so there is really no need to give your pet Reiki every day unless so guided, for they are constantly absorbing love from the vibration of your energy.

You do not need to relearn hand positions or understand the placement of the animal's organs. Simply placing your hands in a location which is pleasing for the animal will allow the light to channel into their bodies. The energy will then go to the place in their little forms which requires care and make the proper changes. If they get up and move away after a few moments of Reiki, realize that they have received all that was needed for that session. Their bodies are small and may need time to adjust to the intensity of the energy. In a short time, they will allow you to administer longer sessions and soon become energy junkies. You will become aware of this as you find these little critters showing up in the room every time

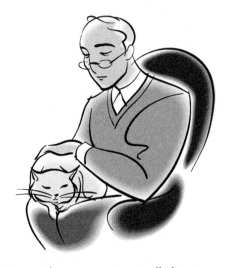

you begin a self-treatment or transfer a healing service to another. My pets actually have adapted quite well to the healing energy in my home and they have learned how to aid in the healing process.

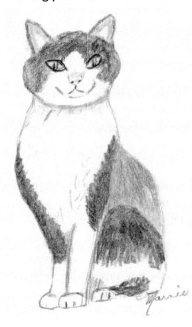

Elliot - 1998 to 2001

Example: For only about three years I was blessed with the presence of a cat who I named Elliot. His name came from the character that played in the movie "ET" and I do think he had some connection to the cosmos as did the boy in the movie. Elliot's sense of when and where to be in a healing session was phenomenal. For some clients he would not wait for them in the treatment room, he would greet them as they entered the driveway. One such client was surprised to find as he turned off the engine of his car that a delightful grey cat had jumped onto the passenger seat to say hello. My client was not alarmed as he told me later he figured, "This must be Marnie's cat." Elliot would greet this man each time he arrived at my home. He just knew what the client's allotted time was and he would show up and help. Elliot did not require an appointment book.

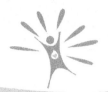

Often Elliot would not appear until the session was just about over; he would then leap onto my massage table and park himself on the feet of my client or nearby. He was adding the finishing touches and grounding the energy so the process would fully integrate.

As pet owners well know, pets do not resonate with all of the guests who come to the home, only the ones who need what they have to offer. Animals naturally have that sixth sense and know who is in need of their care, and they gently respond accordingly. Observe how your animals behave after you have been practicing Reiki. You just may find them assisting in treatments in their own gentle way.

My pet birds also bring in their style of healing. Much of my work is counseling either on the phone or in person. My birds will let me know when I am on track by calling out. Many of my clients hear their chirping and know what was just said requires their added attention. Sometimes it is confirmation and other times they are encouraging us to look deeper into a situation because there is more to be uncovered. A few of my clients will hear my conure's chirping and comment, "Joey agrees." When I am on the phone my birds will not be able to hear the voice of my client but it does not matter, they pick up on the energy and cry out to direct me. It is really quite amusing to observe.

How Pets Carry Negative Energies

When treating a client's pet, always look for similar afflictions that the owner may carry. Pets often carry the physical ailment for their keepers. They serve not only as companions, but healers as well. Be cautious about how this information is presented to the pet's caretaker. One does not want to place blame for the pet's discomfort on their owner. Sending healing light to the owner as well as to the pet will help to transcend any reason for the pet to be ill. Talk to the pet either out loud or silently if guided. Let them know they do not need to injure their body to help their owner. Introduce the animal to the divine assistance which is around their owner. This will release the responsibility the animal feels they have for their beloved owner. Do not have expectations for the results. The energy of Reiki is divinely guided, even in animals. Have a clear intent for the highest and best good to come to all concerned and then let go of the any preconceived ideas for the outcome.

Our furry and feathered friends are also very receptive to distant healing. I have worked very successfully with sheep that I have never touched and have only used distant healing on them. When clearing farm animals, also clear the energy of the buildings and acreage around the animals. The animals protect not only their masters, but also the land where they reside. Look for energy vortices which drain the land. Find gridlines which need reconnecting or water underground which is pulling energy away. You can locate these things by letting your imagination go wild. Anything you perceive could be true on some plane of existence, which is why you thought of it. When you allow images to form in your mind and not push them away, you can easily track the current problems and then the clearing will go much faster.

Example: I was working with a cat that lived on a 25 acre ranch. His owner would bring him for a treatment every week. This little guy was amazing; he would always know when his hour treatment was at an end. He would park himself on the couch and let me administer Reiki to him, but just as the time was running out he would jump up and run around the room.

On one of his visits I tuned into the land around the ranch where he lived. I sensed that an old Native American tribe had lived on this land and I could tell he felt it also. He was protecting their spirits and running their energies through his tiny body. I attuned him to Reiki to show him how he can channel energy. I informed him he could help the spirits by channeling energy to them rather than using his own. I placed symbols into his head and little paws and when I was done, he knew it because up he jumped and this time ran around the entire house. In future treatments I found his energy much clearer and unencumbered by the energies of what he sensed around him.

There are many reasons why an animal may be ill. Be open to the unexpected, trust your instincts and any unusual information you are picking up; then simply ask the problem to clear. It is not always necessary to share all of your perceptions with the owner as you are clearing the animal because not all people are receptive to the information accessed. Know your client and the level of their esoteric beliefs and you will know how much you can share.

Because animals are so receptive to energy, they are also open to communicate with the healers who come to help them. An animal's needs can be sensed quickly and hearing

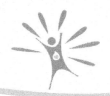

their voice can also become easy with a few simple steps. The first part is to be open to hearing the information and be confident that they will talk to you. You can easily make this connection because you have already adapted this skill. It is similar to listening to the higher self of a client when you are in a session.

Animal Communication

Practicing with an array of different animals, just like working with diverse clients, will quickly increase your ability to pick up silent responses. Start by sitting still with your animal companion, quiet your thoughts and be compassionately present with its spirit. Like making a new friend, you want to let them know you are there for them and interested in what they have to say. Allow this silent relationship to grow and develop like you did when you first met your pet or a

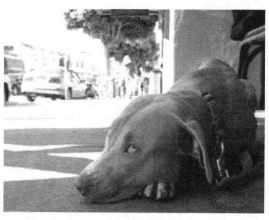

friend's pet. The relationship you are developing acts just like ones you have created with people: some will take to you right away and others will need more time. As you acquire these silent communication skills and release your doubts about talking to animals, you may also find that your ability to intuitively connect with your clients' needs will also improve.

A very important step is to let go of your judgment about your abilities and preconceived ideas you have about your clients, whether they are animals or people. With a little practice, communication from your four-legged friends will become precise and clear. Stop thinking about what they might be saying and observe the animal while you *feel* their response. Accomplishing this goal will be the basis for a good animal communicator. Let go of timeframes, enjoy the moments you are having with the animals, and most of all, just make it fun.

 Remember: Much of the response you will receive will be at first felt, not heard.

Animals are like energetic children: you need to get their attention first before they will talk to you. Recall how you connect with a baby. First you need to make eye contact, softly talk to them and then they will often respond with a smile. Use the same technique with an animal. Make eye contact and then softly speak their name either audibly or in your mind and then listen to what you feel.

Find out if they are ready to listen to you. Are they distracted? If so, move to a location where there is less outside activity. Is this the right time? Maybe they are hungry or tired. To get them to pay attention it may only take a pat on their head or just calling their name so they know you are there. When you are in conversation with another person, you can intuitively tell when someone has not heard what was said. Our response is "Are you listening to me?" It is the same feeling with an animal.

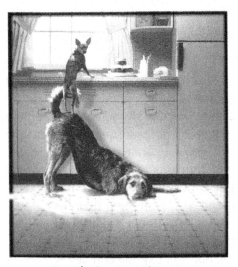

Get their attention

Once you release your fear that this is going to be a difficult task, half of your problems are over. You already hold these abilities to communicate clearly, all you need to do is transfer this knowledge over when you begin to talk with animals.

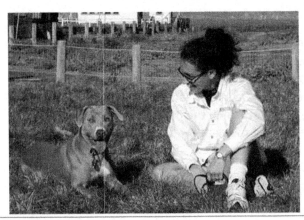

Hold a mental image of the pet talking to you. If you ask for communication but assume it will not happen, the animal is confused and does not know how to respond. Mean what you say and speak with confidence. If this is your animal, they are accustomed to your voice and will find it soothing. Some things are better said in silence, such as issues which may be

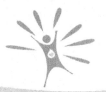

difficult to speak about, like when an animal is having destructive behavior. Don't begin your conversation by pointing out their bad traits. Just like a relationship you have with a person, start the dialogue with non-confrontational speech. By touching the animal and holding them, they will feel assured you have a desire to help. They will pick up that you are not angry at them and that they are safe.

Practice sending mental pictures out, first a few feet in front of your body, then across the room and next to the animal's body. Make this image something they like to do: going for a walk, playing catch at the park, or running and splashing in a stream. What do you sense is their response? Feel the emotion; this is the first way they will connect with you. Let them know you heard them and say thank you. Change the images so that the animal does not get bored with the process and keep the session short. You may always return another day to continue your conversation.

To receive a response from an animal, start with your imagination. Say hello and pretend to hear a reply. Practice with a lot of animals, even ones you pass on the street, just give them a quick silent hello and see if they look at you.

Example: When I am developing a new skill I will immerse myself in the practice for a good month. By concentrating my activities on the application of my new knowledge I will quickly improve these skills and then this new modality will be at my disposal for future reference. I find that I do not have to continue practicing after that one month period because the time was already given to integrate the process into my being and I can draw from it at any time in the future.

The biggest barrier is self-doubt. Know you can pick up information from an animal just like you do when you run your hands over someone's body in a treatment while scanning. Trust the first perceptions you receive because this guidance is instantaneous and transfers quickly. Accept what you are receiving and let the animal know you have heard their answer, say thanks or pat them on the head. Make the sessions short so neither of you becomes frustrated and above all, make it fun. This is an amazing skill. They make movies and TV shows about those who hold these abilities and you too can acquire the talent of an animal whisperer.

Life Tool: Talk to the Animals

1.	Locate a quiet place, away from distracting noises so you will be alone with the animal.
2.	Still your thoughts and lovingly place your attention on the pet as you draw the four traditional Reiki symbols.
3.	Let go of preconceived ideas and judgments about the process and what *should* happen. Leave doubt at the door.
4.	Don't think; open your senses and tune in. What does it feel like to be with this creature? Is it calm, nervous, distracted? What is the vibration in its body?
5.	Get the attention of the animal by looking in its eyes, touching it or speaking its name. Smile at it, feel the response and say thank you.
6.	Send a mental image to the animal of something it likes to do. Send out different images so it does not become bored.
7.	Start with simple, non-invasive questions to establish your new communication skills. Listen, look and feel for the answer and then acknowledge the response.
8.	Ask your question.
9.	Hold a clear image of the animal responding to your questions as you look in its direction or into its eyes. Watch to see what makes it comfortable.
10.	When asking difficult questions, touch or hold the pet if possible.
11.	Accept the reply you receive and acknowledge the response by saying thank you or patting it on the head.
12.	Keep the session short, light and fun.

To find more information about talking to your little friends check out *Animal Reiki* by Elizabeth Fulton and Kathleen Prasad or *Kinship with Animals* by Kate Solisti.

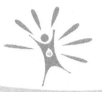

Flower Essence for Animals

When an animal requires assistance to move beyond a stressful situation or memory, flower remedies could prove to be an inexpensive solution. The most common essence to relax an animal is Rescue Remedy by Bach Flower Remedies. It is a combination of plants which have a calming effect on the nervous system of animals as well as people. A few drops of the essence in their water dish or a drop on their paws will do the trick. A common preservative used in most essences is alcohol and this could be harmful to your smaller pets, like birds. You may alleviate this problem by first boiling ¼ cup of water, removing it from the heat and adding five drops of the essence. This will burn off the alcohol. Allow the mixture to cool and then add three drops of the mixture to the bird's water. When working with an essence, note that less is more. The power of the essence builds as the remedy becomes diluted.

Example: Joey is a conure, a small parrot who encouraged me to buy him at a bird show one fall in Denver. When I first went past his cage I noticed him but had no inclination to purchase him. I was looking for a sweet little singing canary. Later I saw a bird flying up in the ceiling of this huge complex. No doubt he had escaped from his

cage. The second time I passed by Joey I was very drawn to him and compelled to purchase him. I did not know it at the time but he was beckoning to me. I brought him home and noticed he was often on the bottom of the cage, which was unusual. Then I saw him fall off his perch and realized he had lost his balance. As I checked his body I found his wings were cut so short that he could not balance and stay on his perch. I had to find out what happened so I made an intuitive inquiry to see what he could tell me about his mishap.

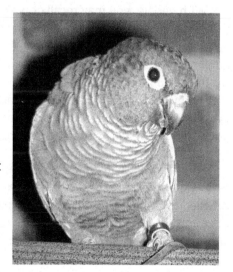

He told me he was the bird who was flying around the complex. He had gotten out of his cage while being shown to a customer and the complex was so large that it took quite some time and effort to catch him. Joey said he had been a very happy bird up until this incident. As he flew around, he was excited to be free and scared all at the same time. He says it was fun. When he was caught, his breeder was so angry he clipped his wings way back as a punishment.

Joey lost not only his trust in people, but his ability to fly. Because of the severity of the clipping, he also lost his balance. He could not even loft down from his perch to the bottom of his cage; he would just fall. I used many remedies over the seven months it took for his feathers to grow back. The essences were not only for stress but also for balance, trauma and fear. The remedies also helped to rebuild Joey's joy. He showed marked improvement with the application of each new remedy.

To find the correct essence for any animal or client, try this procedure: Locate a quiet place and become still and grounded. Connect with the animal and ask which essence they prefer at this time. Using your pendulum, check to see which essence company to start with and then check each individual bottle. I find I can download the healing qualities of the remedies and never even open the bottles. Because remedies are vibrational, they can download into the energy field of the animal or human. This technique allows the bottles to last for a very long time.

With people, you may recall downloading can be achieved by placing the bottle of the essence on the thymus, which is a minor chakra which is located just above the heart. Then ask for the energy of the essence to be transferred into the appropriate bodies - physical, mental, or emotional. For my little bird I placed the bottles he required for the day on the top of his cage and I asked for their frequency to be transmitted into his energy field. Try different approaches to see if you too can manifest results without opening the bottle. And remember that for some, there will still be times when the physical product will need to be ingested.

Some remedy companies are Bach, Perilandra, FES, High Sierra Botanicals or ones you may find at your local health food store or online. Once you find the best essence line, proceed to check each of their products to find the ones which will best serve the needs of your client, two or four legged. Ask how long they need the remedy and then check if another essence is needed after that. I often use Perilandra Essences.

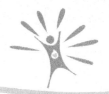

You may find it will not take long to transfer the skills you use with people as a Reiki practitioner, to a very proficient animal communicator. If your intention is pure this talent will be granted. You just may find the animals have a lot to say.

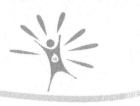

Chapter 9

Beyond Reiki

Even though Reiki has its origin in Japan it holds many Buddhist qualities. We will see how it ties to the steps towards enlightenment which are referenced by the Buddhist monks. They use the physical structure of the stupa (see next page) to reflect this transition. The Reiki symbols are along these steps.

Not only does Reiki follow a path through the body to the spirit realm but there is a direct flow of how it enters the body and finds its way to the physical ailment which is where it is most needed. We will observe this route to better understand this process.

To step beyond the healing attributes of Reiki, the masters must acquaint themselves with the truth of who they are. When a master takes the time to journal their thoughts and feelings from their personality as well as their spirit, much can be obtained. There are exercises which will not take a lot of time but when practiced with consistency will open the channel to higher understandings which for yourself as well as your client. Much of this work will be done in the quantum field of consciousness.

Buddhism and Reiki

When Usui was on his quest to locate information on healing the body, he made inquiries at a Buddhist monastery, knowing that Buddha had the gift of healing. The monks admitted that Buddha and the monks at that time could heal the body and spirit. Over the years the monks had concentrated on only healing the spirit; therefore the knowledge of how to heal the body has been lost. Per the monks' suggestion, Usui ventured up to Mount Kuri Yama and stayed in deep meditation until he as well found the gift to heal.

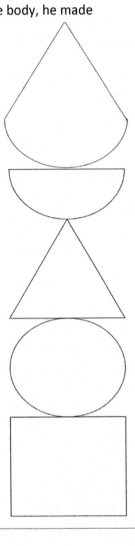

He was happy to find that the symbols and energy he was given reflected the healing of not only the body, but the spirit as well, thus creating a connection from Reiki to Buddhism. The tie between these two practices can be seen reflected in the stupa. The stupa is a sacred building which often holds a relic of the Buddha and is constructed for prayer and meditation. As we look at the Reiki symbols and their meanings you will see how both carry the steps to enlightenment. The symbols and levels of Reiki are constructed the same way as the stupa. This will show how the spirit is lifted along its journey to enlightenment.

The stupa consists of five geometric shapes: the square, the circle, the triangle, the half circle and the Cintamani, which holds the form of a jewel. At the bottom of the stupa is the square. It creates a solid base on the earth while it honors and points in the four sacred directions. Like Cho-Ku-Rei, it is grounding and the focus is physical. The similarities between this section of the stupa and Cho-Ku-Rei are clearing through

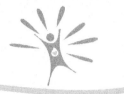

the physical, which was created in the initial awakening during the first Reiki attunement. Cho-Ku-Rei, like the base of the stupa, anchors one to solid ground.

The circle is connected with Sei-He-Ki; it tunes into the emotional body. The element of this part of the stupa is water, which reflects emotions, as does Sei-He-Ki, the mental and emotional symbol. Practice is required in second degree Reiki in order to memorize this level's complicated symbols. As the symbols are rehearsed, they are integrated into the life style of the practitioner, which completes a circle of energy.

In the triangle, Hon-Sha-Ze-Sho-Nen equates to the mind and the mental body. Hon-Sha-Ze-Sho-Nen has no healing qualities of its own; it does no more than move the Reiki energy though space and time. It is a chariot which is driven only by the mind. The intent of thought directs Reiki to someone miles away, into the past, or to a future event. The practitioner must quiet their mind and clearly imagine the time, place and location of the future or past situation. The physical body of the healer does not changed location; all movement is in the mind. As one moves up the stupa towards enlightenment, the mind must be cleared of outside chatter. Therefore, this higher level represents the silencing of the idle talk within the mind which will then empower any intent set forth by the master.

The next step up the stupa is the half circle, it holds the spiritual body and is tied to Dai-Ko-Myo, the master symbol. The image here reflects the opening to the divine above which cradles the master energy. Because this is a half circle rather than a full circle it is fully open to all which can be received from above. Via the opening which occurs in the master attunement, the student can now quickly enter into a deeper state of meditation which will intensify the senses, bringing the student closer to nirvana. As all of the five senses - sight, smell, taste, hearing and touch- are opened, and intuition is greatly increased. The five senses are the bodily activities which keep the master grounded and in present time. When healers leave their body when giving a treatment, they diminish the intensity of the healing practice; there lays the importance of being aware of the body though the five senses and staying in contact with them at all times.

The master level of Reiki will generate a soul-to-soul connection from the healer to the client. In the beginning levels of Reiki, the energy is channeled from the higher self of the practitioner into the bodies of the client, where it is directed by their higher self to the location where they require healing. The master is actually working from their spirit to the client's spirit, which gives the ability to perform spiritual counseling and deeper healing. Dai-Ko-Myo represents this soul-to-soul connection and here at the half circle in the stupa, the spiritual body is enveloped with divine love and also linked to it.

The top of the stupa holds the Cintamani. In Hinduism and Buddhism, it is a magical jewel which holds the power of manifestation. It is attained by the Buddhas and Bodhisattvas, who are the beings who have stepped into full enlightenment. Raku is the master teacher symbol which passes on Reiki wisdom to others, therefore, the highest step. The enlightenment brought forth from the Universe into the body is awakening the light within the body. At the top of the stupa is the representation of the jewel of enlightenment which ties to the jewel of light the master teacher esoterically hands to each student during attunements. Diane Stein, in *Essential Reiki,* draws the connection of the Buddhist "raising of the soul" to Reiki and its symbols in the following chart.

The Stupa and Steps to Enlightenment

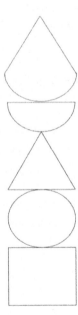

Raku
    Enlightenment
    Soul
Dai-Ko-Myo
    Spiritual Body
Hon-Sha-Ze-Sho-Nen
    Mind
    Mental Body
Sai-He-Kei
    Practice
    Emotional Body
Cho-Ku-Rei
    Original Awakening
    Physical Body

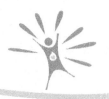

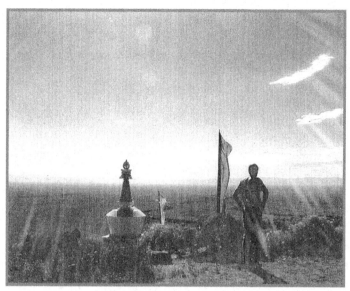

View of the top of the stupa overlooking
the valley in Crestone, Colorado

The Path of Reiki

Reiki, when consciously directed, will flow from the Universe into the head, heart and hands of the practitioner and to the client. The energy is directed to where there is the greatest need. The practitioners hands could be on the head of the client, yet the vibration can be felt in the back where there has been chronic pain. The mystery of how energy travels to where it needs to be can be explained by the following path.

As the energy enters the body it will flow first into the chakras, then to the secondary energy pathways called the nadis, and from those etheric nerves it enters into the physical nervous system. Next to be approached with this divine light are the organs held within the endocrine system and then it channels into the blood. From that point the higher self will send the energy to the place it is most needed in the body.

Nadis are not physical but they take a form similar to that of physical things such as electrical conduits, nerves, veins, vessels or arteries. They can be envisioned as a web of light that rests in the body's aura. It holds the composition of the subtle body which channels the flow of the unseen vital life force or prana.

These tiny fibers direct the energy into the meridian lines and then into the nervous system. Meridian lines are found in Chinese medicine and are energy highways where acupressure points lie. Nadis can also be understood to be a light web which also encompasses the axiatonal lines referenced in the *Keys of Enoch* (chapter 3-1-7.) Axiatonal lines are part of our light body and can be felt, intuitively read and realigned. They are a subset of the meridian lines. This light body activation is taught through Light Internal and is often the next step after learning Reiki.

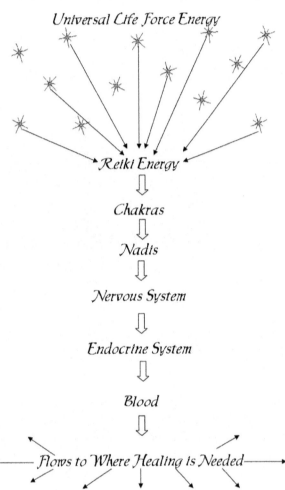

The Path of Reiki into the Body

Universal Life Force Energy

Reiki Energy

⇓

Chakras

⇓

Nadis

⇓

Nervous System

⇓

Endocrine System

⇓

Blood

⇓

Flows to Where Healing is Needed

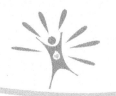

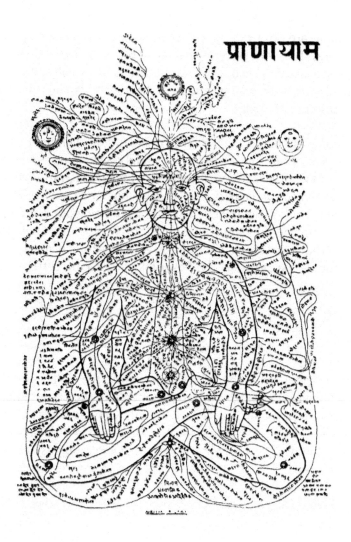

प्राणायाम

Nadis

The above illustration is from David V. Tansley, *Subtle Body - Essence and Shadow*, (1977, Art and Imagination Series, Thames and Hudson, London). In that book this illustration is labeled "The nadis, diagram, Tibet," but the writing is Sanskrit, not Tibetan, and both the artistic style and also the arrangement of the chakras is Indian.

All healing modalities are similar in the fact that they use the same channels of the body to direct the energy. Different systems use varied terminology, but the results are often the same. Having a visual focus of this information highway will assist the practitioner to mentally direct the energy, although the flow is actually happening automatically and faster than thought.

The body is one complete unit, a web of light connected through the meridian lines, acupressure points and axiatonal lines. The organs, endocrine glands, nerves and blood vessels are part of this molecular highway. Placement of the hands varies with each individual; following your intuitive guidance will always supersede published hand positions. There are times when the hands will be drawn to hold opposite areas of the body. Touching the left hip and the right shoulder at the same time will balance the flow within the light grid of the body. When you listen to your inner voice and allow your hands to move without mental direction, the flow of healing can be better sensed.

Journaling

One of the steps on the rungs of the ladder to mastery is the ability to truly know one's self. Not the self which was molded from childhood into the predesigned form of society or family values. Here you are looking for the self who has for years tried to be seen, understood and loved. One of the best ways to know and understand this aspect of yourself is to jot down some of your personal as well as divine thoughts each day. It does not have to be for the eyes of anyone else but you may write as though it is.

Express what you would like others to know about your dreams, joys, accomplishments and deeply held emotions. What do you secretly hold within yourself, hoping no one will discover it or perhaps wishing that they would? If your innermost thoughts were exposed, what do you think would happen to you? What are your deepest fears? All of these questions can be answered by taking time to express your thoughts with a pen and paper or on a computer. In these private moments, you will understand why you act the way you do with others, as well as why you think the thoughts that form in your mind. From these steps you can begin to know and love yourself, just as you are, without any changes or reasons to be different. Once you entertain the idea that you are perfect just the way you are you will hold the gift to open others to do the same.

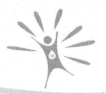

When you set pen to paper observe who is writing. Is it your inner child, adolescent, adult or higher self? Each of these characters needs time to speak and express their feelings. Ultimately the adult and higher self will prevail, but not until all aspects of the self are given their place on center stage. Once you become familiar with these parts of yourself, their voices and how they perform, you will know which ones are presenting themselves when you are interacting with others on a daily basis. The value is when you can acknowledge their presence but know there is no need to allow them to run the show. This diminishes their power and puts the adult back in charge.

Life is not perfect. Each experience and assumed mistake has an underlying purpose which can come out in the open, during journaling. This knowledge will release judgments, create a space of self-acceptance and expand your heart.

One way to know who is speaking through your writing is to give them different colored pens with which to write. Have one color, perhaps purple, for your higher self, blue for your own thoughts, green for your adolescent and red for your inner child. When you begin to write with your purple pen, start your statement as if your angel was standing before you and then entering your thoughts. Would it not express adoration and love for you? At first pretend to record the thoughts of this being by making things up and have the correspondence very positive.

Example: When writing from your divine essence begin in this way:
Good morning, light being, I am part of your royal family and we are always very proud of you. We are here at all times; there is no need for you to feel alone or without guidance. If you have any questions at all you may ask any of us and we will do our best to fully answer your questions. Take a moment, put down your pen and feel my love. Once you can fully sense my presence then pick up your pen and begin to write once again. I love you.

Journaling can be a way to clear former issues which are locked away in the subconscious mind. To access this part of your psyche do not judge what you are writing, just write. Often what you are writing appears repetitive but after reading it later, you will find it will make more sense. When you read what you wrote days later notice if the words seem familiar or does it seem like someone else was writing? I find when I reread my journal weeks later, looking back at what I wrote, it all seems new to me, and that is my clue there was another part of my presence writing, for these words do not reflect my conscious mind.

The practice of journaling is similar to meditation only more active. Follow the same steps you use for meditation by writing when you will be undisturbed, and you definitely at a time you are not feeling rushed. On the days you need a pick me up, you may find it comforting to write from your higher self and receive compliments and adoration. There are many ways to journal, you can:

- Channel your angel.
- Ask for guidance from your higher self.
- Propose a question.
- Look at information from your dreams.
- Just have fun with automatic writing.

Another way to access information is automatic writing. It is a similar to how you connect with spirits on the other side. First you will find a constructive spirit to talk with and then let their energy move your pen. This practice is fun because as you let go your hand will surprisingly move with no direction from your conscious mind. This practice is a new venture you both you and the spirit. The spirit is learning how to connect in this physical way which is a new activity for them, so be patient and let the process unfold for the weeks that you are communicating with this entity. Keep in mind you want to ask for the same spirit each time you sit down to write.

 Remember: Always ask for a spirit with powers and knowledge equal to or greater than your own.

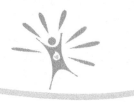

Life Tool: Journaling

Before you begin close your eyes and drop into the center of your being.
Perhaps this will be your heart or an un-described place which can only be felt.

1.	Write at a time when you will be undisturbed, locate a quiet place and begin to still your mind.
a.	Before retiring for the night your guides will often talk to you just as you fall asleep. Keep a paper and pen by your bed.
b.	They will also communicate the moment you awake, while you are still in a semi-dream state.
c.	Buddhists find 3 AM is the best time to connect with spirit.
2.	Use two colored pens, a blue one for personal thoughts and a purple one for your higher essence, angel or guide.
3.	Start with your blue pen and just write about your day.
4.	Now switch to your purple pen.
5.	Begin with an adoring salutation. This will prime the pump of your imagination and get you rolling.
a.	Your angelic presence addresses you with respect and love for example: Blessed being of light, Hello special one, Greetings star traveler.
b.	This is all in your imagination until it becomes reality, so have fun with it.
6.	Let the words flow. Start with praising yourself for what you have done lately.
a.	This will make a connection to your guide.
b.	Soon the words will begin to flow.
c.	Write what you wish someone would say to you. Soon you will find things will begin to form in your mind which you did not make up.
7.	Do not judge or edit what you are writing. It will look different when you read it at a later date.
8.	Fake it till you make it and most of enjoy what you are doing.
9.	When you become proficient with receiving information from your angelic self you may begin to write angel messages for your clients. This is a very nice way to end a healing treatment.

Life Tool: Dream Journal

1.	Before you go to sleep tell yourself, I will remember my dreams and/or I ask to meet my spirit guides.
2.	Do this for a period of one week and only ask for the connection, no more.
3.	After one week, you may ask for an answer to a question.
4.	Write your question in your journal before you go to sleep.
5.	Immediately upon awakening write your answer in the journal. The message is more accessible when you are still drowsy.
6.	Record images or thoughts if you are awakened in the night. To stay in a semi-dream state, don't even turn on the lights. This information can come in as metaphors which will make sense later.
7.	It could take three days to get an answer, so be patient.
8.	You may also request for clarity of your dreams. Jot down your visions as soon as you wake up because the memory fades quickly.
9.	The understanding of a dream may come to you during the day while you are doing mindless work. Watch for the information and pay attention to metaphors.
10.	You may try your hand at lucid dreaming; this is when you inner act with your dreams. You are aware of dreaming and can consciously change what is occurring in the dream. This is a fun one.
11.	As you retire for the night affirm I will be lucid and become conscious in my dreams tonight. Give this a few days and then you will see the results.

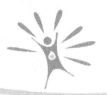

 Life Tool: Automatic Writing

1.	Take a few minutes to still your mind and body by taking three deep breaths, relax your muscles from head to toe and open your chakras one at a time.
2.	Make the intent to connect to a constructive being that has knowledge equal to or greater than yours. You may also ask for one who has specific information about a problem or situation.
3.	As their energy moves in to move the pen you may sense a shift. Your body could jerk or there may be a temperature change. Observe and pay attention.
4.	Hold a pen loosely in your hand. Let the pen move; do not try to move it yourself. You may begin the process by scribbling then, watch as words will begin to form.
5.	The being on the other side is also practicing; it is trying to figure out how to move your pen, so support this being in its adventures.
6.	It may start out as gibberish, let it be; a message will eventually come through.
7.	Remember when you are being creative the last thing you want is someone telling you that is does not make sense, this guide just might feel the same way.
8.	Do not second guess what you are writing, this will stop the flow. It may take a few sessions to get a comprehendible message.
9.	Give yourself and the spirit being, time to understand how the two of you can best open to your communications.
10.	Once you perfect this skill you may write messages for other people.

Life Tool: Conscious Writing

1.	Write down a question or describe where you need assistance or guidance.
2.	Sit comfortably and signal your body to relax by taking three deep breaths.
3.	Place the question in a bubble, do not try to solve the question, just let it float in a field of light before your eyes.
4.	Allow the request to drop into the quantum field of no space and no time. Sit within this space until you once again become somewhat conscious.
5.	Then pick up your pen and begin a stream of writing.
	a. Write anything that comes into your thoughts.
	b. Do not edit your thinking.
6.	Your thoughts may start with nonsense. Just let it flow: it will change over time and begin to make sense.

 Life Tool: Walking with Your Angels

1.	Set the intent to be conscious of your angels in any form.
2.	Before leaving for work sit quietly for two to five minutes either in your car or in your house.
	a. Imagine an open a door in your energy field which is a divine portal and welcome in a divine light being.
	b. Notice if you feel any sensations in or outside of your body. There may be a breeze, a warm feeling all over or a brush on your face.
	c. These sensations can be very subtle so watch for them.
3.	On the drive to work notice how many courtesies are directed your way. Who lets you cut in front of them or smiles as you pass by.
4.	Pay attention to strangers at lunch, phone conversations, words you hear as you pass by people, music on the radio and even confrontations.
	a. Your angels may be people you already have had contact with or a person who has briefly passed by. Just pay attention.
	b. Confrontations may bring their own divine messages.

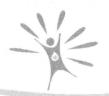

	c. Often the person who gives you a message from your angel will not recall saying it, days later.
5.	Watch for the ways your angels contact you. They are clever and have a wonderful sense of humor.
6.	Angelic directives are accessed in various ways:
	a. Media; radio, TV, billboards, music.
	b. Conversations that are not directed at you but you overhear.
7.	Practice this exercise for three days.
8.	Your angels will be contacting you. Open your inner eyes; look, listen.
9.	Be grateful each day even if you have noticed nothing, as gratitude will enhance the process. The days that you feel you have received the least are often the days that you have obtained the most.

Stepping into the Quantum Field

When channeling Reiki or while meditating you move into a place which scientists call the quantum field. There is a sensation felt which is often difficult to describe yet you know you have slipped out of third-dimensional reality and into a deeper space. This happens naturally just by requesting Reiki to flow but there is more that can be accomplished in this zone with a minimum amount of effort.

You may find it fun to practice working within the quantum field and observing the results. By dropping into this place you are stepping into a space of unlimited possibilities. Here there are no agenda, no steps to follow and no rules. You can place a desire into this field and then step into present time and merely feel what changes occur. Dr. Richard Bartlett, author of *Matrix Energetics,* expands on this concept and how he steps into this field to assist himself and others.

Dr. Deepak Chopra authored numerous books which clearly show how the medical community is unknowingly tied to metaphysics, through a quantum level of existence. As we look within the minute aspects of the body, the spaces revealed between the molecules of the cells are far more vast than we can imagine. Moving deeper into this quantum field, the space appears so expanded that it can be observed as more space between the molecules than there are molecules themselves, making us more space than matter.

As we view these tiny particles are viewed, they mimic the universe and are as separate from each other as the distance of a star from a planet. So, as energy is directed deeper into the body, the cosmos is revealed, reflecting the Universal life force, which is being channeled into the physical form through various healing practices, one of which is Reiki.

As the higher spiritual levels are channeled through a healing modality into the client, the healing force flows into the core quantum level of their bodies and when that occurs, the energy moves out into the universe once again. Energy will seek its own likeness, so it finds this similarity within the body and expands it. Once this expansion occurs, what was out of balance in the body dissolves into the pure divine space held in the divine Universe. This is how healing can occur in the physical, mental or emotional body of a person within an instant.

When I work with a physical ailment, emotional distress, unwanted spirit forms or anything which is hindering an individual from the beautiful light being which they are, I work in this expanded quantum field. When I acknowledge that this is the only energy in existence, the form will balance and the individual will sense the difference.

The intensity of this expansion needs to be connected to the earth through the body. We are earth-bound beings and are required to stay on the planet in mind and body. Even though one is channeling cosmic light, a solid anchor is required to heal and balance the energy for the client. This is called grounding and a necessary part of the any transformational process.

Grounding is a natural process which is shown in the chemistry of the body. Every element in the earth can be found within the physical form. So, connecting to the earth is bringing the body back to its origin. In like form, the light, through drawn from the cosmos, also exists within the body and that too is being reclaimed.

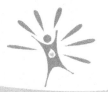

You must create time to be alone in order to connect to your gifts. As long as others are present either physically, emotionally, mentally or spiritually you are under their influence. On a physical level you need to clear their energy fields to make a space for the stillness to reside. By doing this you will open to find your truth uninfluenced by the opinions of family and friends. You need to make a decision need and it often becomes automatic to respond in a way which is accepted by those around you, giving little attention to the quiet thoughts within your mind.

Those are the whispers which are softly in the distance of your mind are your spiritual inner trying to get your attention. It cannot be heard until you silence the outside voices around you. When you do not follow this directive the Universe will make the decision for you. This comes in the form of losing a job which you have wanted to leave for months, or a relationship dissolving before your very eyes, yet you have wanted out of it for some time. All these appear to be outside forces arranging your life but the truth of the matter is you have created it and put it into action. It is a lot less stressful if you consciously become aware of what you are doing subconsciously and then act on it from your conscious mind.

Example: I know when the Universe is pushing me into these silent. I will pick up the phone and begin to call friends only to find no one is home. The ones who answer do not have time to see me. It is for my own good but I do resist. At first I am frustrated and want my own way. I want companionship. As I give into the inevitable, I relax in the stillness and enjoy my time with the company of myself. Then I find it turns out to be quite a pleasant period. These are times I am not looking for messages or answers, these are just times to be still.

~ *I want to know if you can be alone with yourself and*

if you truly like the company you keep in the empty moments. ~

Oriah Mountain Dreamer

As you advance, you too will find this space will automatically be created for you. There is no need to send your friends away; they will leave all on their own. There will be a point when no one is available for a quick lunch or a quiet dinner. There will be days when each person you call will not answer the phone; this is a sign that it is time to go within. Sit in the silence and let it envelop each of your senses. Do not attempt to appease the feeling of separation by turning on the television, watching a movie or listening to your favorite music. These quiet moments are reflected best as the sun sets and the house becomes dark. If you sit still the entire home will begin to have a calming presence which cannot be found when others are around. This becomes a gift you give yourself.

Applying Reiki in all Aspects of Life

The techniques and ideas presented in this book can assist you in all aspects of your life. When pain arises in yourself or others, you can ease it. When stressed, you can calm your emotions. You perhaps have even seen how you can apply this channeled energy of love into inanimate objects like computers, traffic, or business meetings. The applications are endless. This is now the time for you to design how you will use this channeled energy of love to help yourself and others in your work life.

Example: Greg is a **manager** in a plumbing company and he could not see how Reiki could help him at work. His comment was, "I do not place my hands on people like a massage therapist, so why would knowing how to channel energy help me?" The answer is simple; when people need a plumber they usually are stressed. The water damage which can occur from broken pipes and leaking toilets needs quick attention and scheduling immediate help is not always possible. When Greg talks to a customer on the phone if their problem is not remedied in the proper time desired by the customer, they often become irate. This negative energy is directed to Greg and in the past he took it on and held onto it even when he returned home in the evening. This became very stressful for him and his family.

Words only suffice up to a point; these customers needed something to ease their agitation. Greg applied the process he learned in class by imagining violet light entering his head and allowing it to not only come through his hands into the phone line but also energetically flow out of his voice. The calming energy of Reiki was then

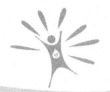

sent through his voice to the customer. He found the person at the other end of the line would become calm and open to accepting the schedule he was presenting to them.

Sue is a **respiratory therapist** who found that applying Reiki to herself a few times a week allowed her to be calmer during the stress of her day. Often she would be called over the intercom to assist a patient who had gone into trauma and needed her care right away. In the past she would run down the hall filling her mind with various scenarios about what she would need to do if ... All this chatter within her mind was stressful and consumed her energy. The "what if" stories running in her mind were cluttering her thoughts and using excessive energy, making her exhausted at the end of the day.

After learning to channel the energy of Reiki, Sue found when she was paged, she still hurried to assist the patients in distress but now her mind was silent, there was no dialogue running about what would need to be done. Sue found when she arrived at the patient's side, her thoughts were clear; she knew exactly what to do and how to proceed. Because she learned how to release the unnecessary chatter and stress in her mind she found her days would go smoothly and she would have more energy at the end of her day when she returned home.

Sharon is a prima **ballerina** who knows how to radiate her spiritual presence during her performance. Other dancers would watch her in the wings, wondering what she was doing before she entered the stage. Why did she stand in silence before stepping into the lights? Sharon would take just a moment to connect to her higher self and balance her energies, and only then would she enter the stage. Once on stage she told me, she would direct her light energy all the way to the back rows of the auditorium.

The audience would applaud as she appeared but they were not only reacting to her obvious talent and charisma, they were responding to the divine energy she was projecting. Unknown to the audience they were affected by what she brought to the stage in the form of her "presence." This is an energy she had honed into a fine talent.

Terry worked in the **corporate world** where she used the energy of Reiki and the knowledge she learned about chakras to help her in business meetings while she was in her busy corporate environment. She would sit in a meeting and rather than becoming agitated because ideas were being presented had no point or target, she found she could make a difference. Terry would imagine a focus of light from the Universe flowing into the center of the room, rushing over the table, papers and those who sat in the chairs. Soon a calm presence would come over the room, presenters would get back on track and much would be accomplished in a very short period of time.

When one business associate would try to push a point Terry would send energy from her third eye into theirs and then listen to their inner voice. She would then be able to hear their point of view, not from their physical voice but from an inner understanding she was intuitively picking up. Terry could then respond appropriately, releasing the tension caused by the person who was being misunderstood.

When people become irritated at meetings it is only because they feel no one hears them, so they say the same thing louder or with malice in their voice. Channeling Reiki energy which is actually love, in their direction, and tuning into their intuitive chakra changes the whole situation. No hands are placed on their body but they will feel the shift and respond positively.

As you can see, there is no limit to how channeling love into the work environment can make the day a lot more pleasant. Reiki is not only to be applied when you get home and relax, but it can naturally be a part of your day. It becomes fun to see how others react when love is directed to them. This then becomes a life style, rather than a practice.

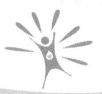

Cleansing Journal

Using the journal will keep the student aware of their rising vibration in each of the four bodies and all seven chakras. It will assist to ground the incoming light and to keep them in the present time. Make the memoranda short to encourage and support the process each day.

Day   1   Chakra 1

_____
_____
_____
_____
_____
_____
_____

Day   2   Chakra 2

_____
_____
_____
_____
_____
_____

Day   3   Chakra 3

_____
_____
_____
_____
_____
_____
_____

Day   4   Chakra 4

_____
_____
_____
_____
_____
_____

Day   5   Chakra 5

_____
_____
_____
_____
_____
_____

Day   6   Chakra 6

_____
_____
_____
_____
_____

Day   7   Chakra 7

_____
_____
_____
_____
_____
_____

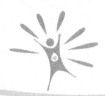

Day 8   Chakra 1

_____
_____
_____
_____
_____
_____

Day 9   Chakra 2

_____
_____
_____
_____
_____

Day 10   Chakra 3

_____
_____
_____
_____
_____
_____

Day 11   Chakra 4

_____
_____
_____
_____
_____
_____

Day 12   Chakra 5

_____
_____
_____
_____
_____
_____
_____
_____

Day 13   Chakra 6

_____
_____
_____
_____
_____
_____
_____

Day 14   Chakra 7

_____
_____
_____
_____
_____
_____
_____

Day 15   Chakra 1

_____
_____
_____
_____
_____
_____
_____

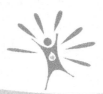

Day 16   Chakra 2

_____
_____
_____
_____
_____
_____

Day 17   Chakra 3

_____
_____
_____
_____
_____
_____

Day 18   Chakra 4

_____
_____
_____
_____
_____
_____

Day 19   Chakra 5

_____
_____
_____
_____
_____
_____
_____
_____

Day 20   Chakra 6

_____
_____
_____
_____
_____

Day 21   Chakra 7

_____
_____
_____
_____
_____
_____

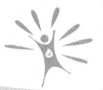

Afterword

Now that you have practiced the exercises on yourself and others it is time to move on. None of the examples presented in this book were meant to be set in stone. They are to support you as a master while you develop your individual techniques. Through practice you will begin to uncover and claim your personal approach which awakens the gifts which are held within. No one can find it for you; no one can direct you to this, for this is your inner search and, at times, a solitary one. Step into your power as a master and know you can now obtain information which has not been accessed on this planet before. My hope for you is that as you explore the healing styles of those who have gone before you, you can then see how you can create your own method.

Claim your inner power by questioning the unusual and obtaining your own answers. When a system appears to be out of sync with the norm but you sense there is no problem, honor the information you are being given. This is the mark of a master.

To truly become master of your life, you must first know yourself. This is easier said than done, for it takes a lifetime for the truth of who you are to unfold. Just when you think you have figured it out, a new element appears. As people enter and reenter your life, new aspects of yourself are revealed. Each person who blesses you with their presence carries with them reflections of you, both complimentary and negative. Look with unsuspecting eyes and be compassionate towards others and this will naturally bring into your being, a sense of self love. The process of walking life's path is to accept ourselves as we are.

~ Know thyself and the truth shall set you free ~
Socrates

The power which lies within each of us has a sense of flow. It cannot be directed, controlled or given, it is only felt. All of our bodies try to figure out this power but there is no way to actually do that. The mental body analyzes, the emotional body obsesses, the physical body resists as the spiritual body tries to claim ownership. The illusion can be broken when you take time to detach from these false impressions and sit in the emptiness. Then your individual truth will surface and can be acknowledged.

A master selects their own path, from their personal guidance found within their heart. No one can tell you what your destination is on this adventure. Keep in mind that it is the journey, not the destination, which matters. Others may guide you and reveal clues along the way, but you are the one who will uncover the mysteries which will open your heart and then you may show others how to do the same. It can be a path of pain and frustration, or a walk of thrill and adventure. You select the process and the experience. Every step is yours to take; the rest of your life starts today. May you embark on your journey in love.

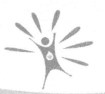

Appendix

Auras by Mark Smith: Exercises to open inner sight to see auras in only 60 seconds.

Love is in the Earth by Melody: An array of information about crystals and gems. Lists ailments, numerology, zodiac relations and much more.

Love is in the Earth, Laying-on-of-Stones by Melody: Comprehensive exercises to experience the power of crystals when placed in geometric shapes around the body.

The Healer's Manual by Ted Andrews: A good overview on various healing techniques; also covers how to make gemstone elixirs.

Reiki with Gemstones by Klingger-Omenka: As the title implies, it gives ways to work with stones and Reiki.

Reiki and Other Rays of Healing Touch by Katheen Ann Milner: An extensive inventory of symbols from Reiki and other healing modalities.

Wheel of Life by Anodea Judith: An advanced approach in explaining the chakra system, along with physical exercises to open and clear the chakras.

Reiki Fire by Frank Arjava Petter: A different view of the history of Reiki. Petter traveled to Japan and uncovered new information.

Notes

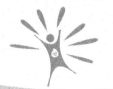

Notes

Bibliography

Bartlett, Richard, D.C., N.D. *Matrix Energetics.* Hillsboro OR: Beyond Words, 2007

Brennan, Barbara. *Hand of Light.* New York, NY: Bantam Books, 1998

Brown, Dan. *The Da Vinci Codes. New York,* NY: Double Day, 2003

Dale, Cyndi. *The Complete Book of Chakra Healing.* St. Paul MI: Llewellyn, 1996

Fulton, Elizabeth & Prasad, Kathleen. *Animal Reiki.* Berkley CA: Ulysses Press, 2006

Hay, Louise. *Heal Your Body.* Carson, CA: Hay House, Inc., 1982

Hurtak, J.J. *Keys of Enoch.* Los Gatos, *CA:* The Academy for Future Science, 1997

Melody. *Love is in the Earth.* Wheat Ridge, CO: Earth-Love Publishing House, 1995

Melody, *Love is in the Earth: Laying-on-of-Stones.* Wheat Ridge, CO: Earth-Love Publishing House, 1991

Solisti, Kate & Tobias, Michael. Kinship with Animals. San Francisco, CA: Council Oak Books, 2006

Stein, Diane. *Essential Reiki.* Marshall MN: The Crossings Press, 1997

Truman, Karol. *Feelings Buried Alive Never Die.* St. George, UT: Olympus Distributing, 1991

Wright, Michell Small. *Map, The Co-Creative White Brotherhood Medical Assistance Program.* Warrenton VA: Perelendra LTD, 1990

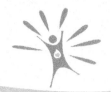

Index

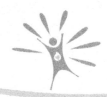

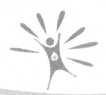

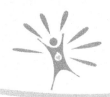

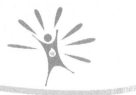

About the Author

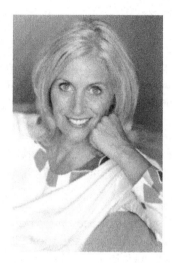

Marnie Vincolisi has been lecturing on Reiki, metaphysics, spiritual growth for decades. The classes she has developed are on subjects as varied as divination, space clearing, ear coning, sacred geometry, meditation and ascended masters. Marnie currently lives in the Southwestern United States. She travels to lecture and gives attunements and treatments remotely. Her treatments are for optimal health, emotional balance, mental clarity and spiritual connection.

Marnie's books, meditation CDs and MP3s may be found at
www.lightinternal.com
You may contact Marnie for personal sessions at
marnie@lightinternal.com

Presentation slides to support the study of Reiki, graphically illustrate the methods presented in this and other books by Marnie Vincolisi. The slides are suitable for class presentations and are available at www.lightinternal.com

Finding Your Inner Gift, the Ultimate Reiki 1st Degree Manual
Inner Gifts Uncovered, the Complete Reiki 2nd Degree Manual
Claiming Your Inner Gifts, the Comprehensive Study of Master Reiki

The House Who Found Its Home
A delightful children's book about a house that is not happy with where it lives. It was too tight, too bright and too noisy! So the house took off to find a new place to live. As it journeyed to new places it found many adventures along the way and discovered a valuable lesson.

Meditation Made Easy and *Cosmic Connections* feature the melodic voice of Marnie Vincolisi in CD format. The CDs may be used for understanding our chakra systems through guided imagery meditation and for meditations during the attunement process for Reiki Master Teachers. Also found on *Meditation Made Easy* is the process for a Reiki self-treatment, easily guided by Marnie, each available as a CD or an MP3 online at www.lightinternal.com

CPSIA information can be obtained
at www.ICGtesting.com
Printed in the USA
LVOW04s2027180517

535011LV00004B/278/P